AF790633

Recent Advances in Digital System Diagnosis and Management of Healthcare

Edited by Kamran Sartipi and Thierry Edoh

Published in London, United Kingdom

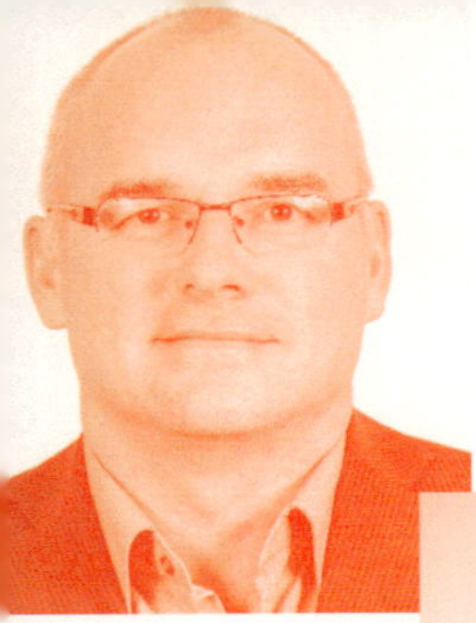
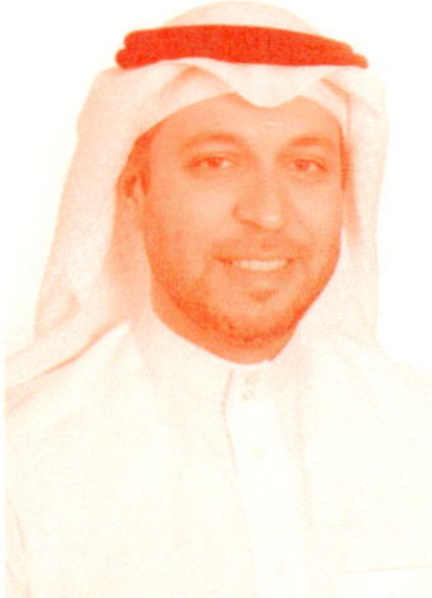
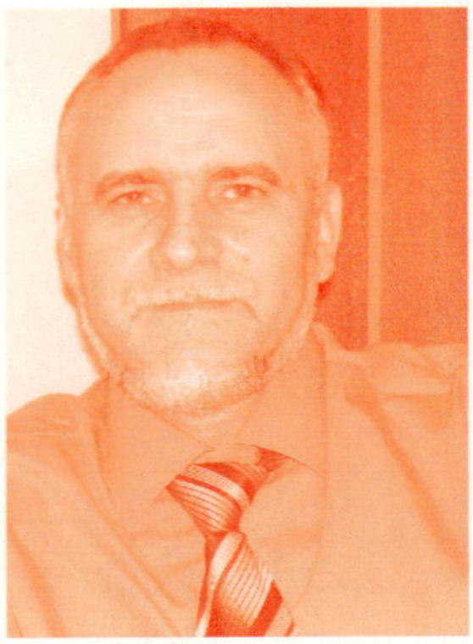
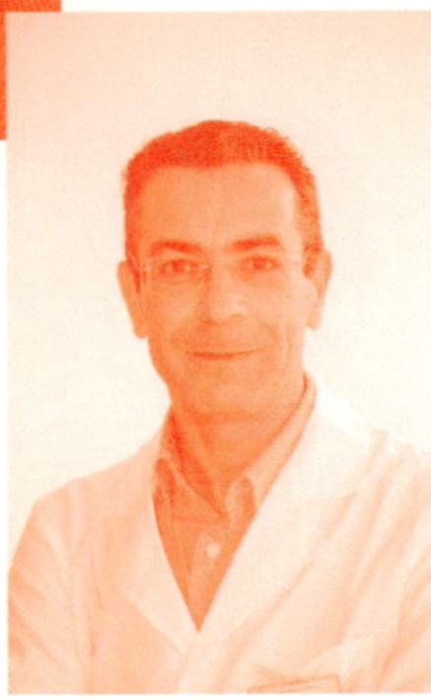
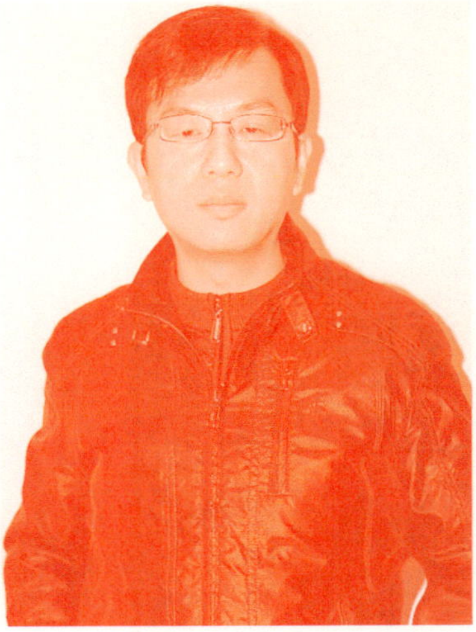
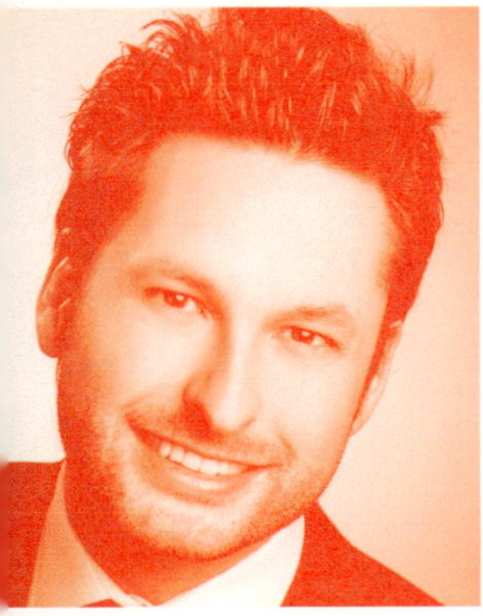
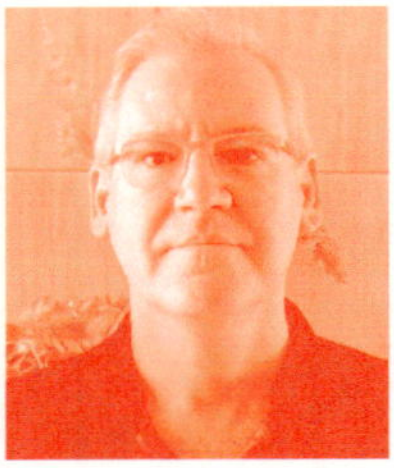

IntechOpen

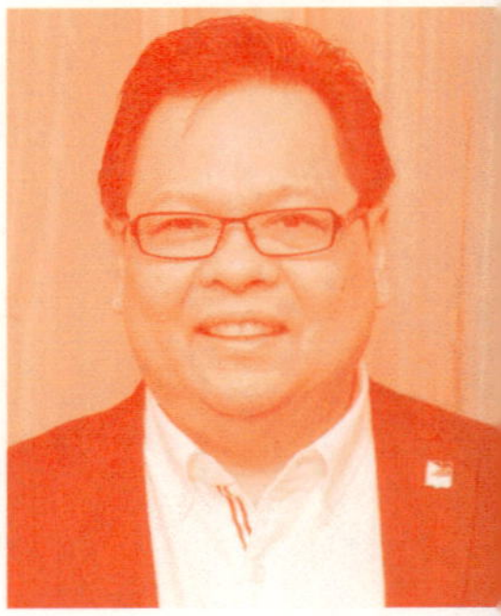
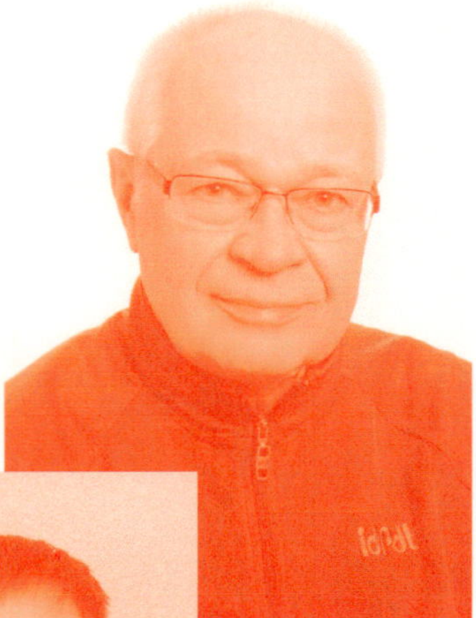
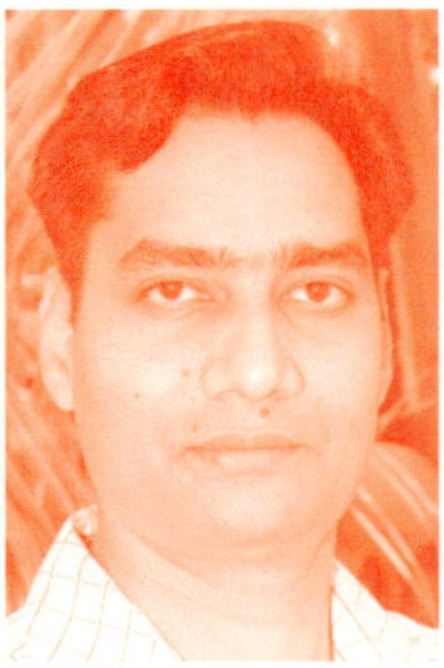
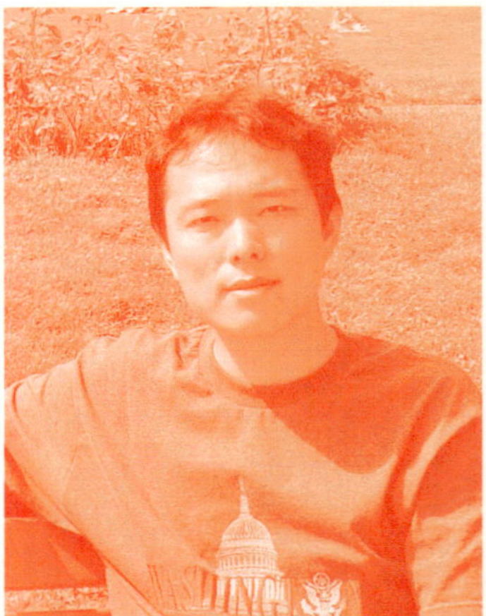
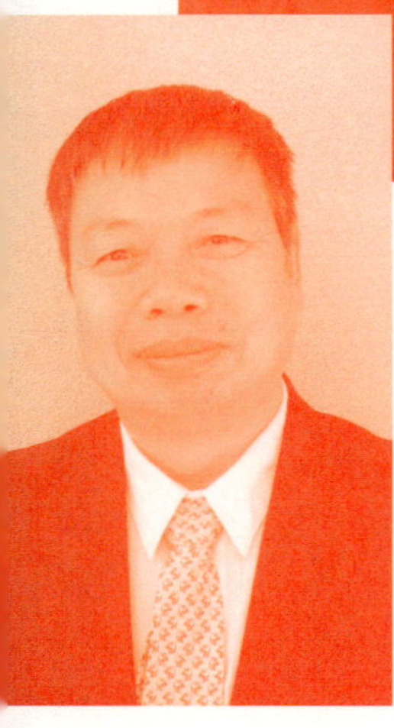
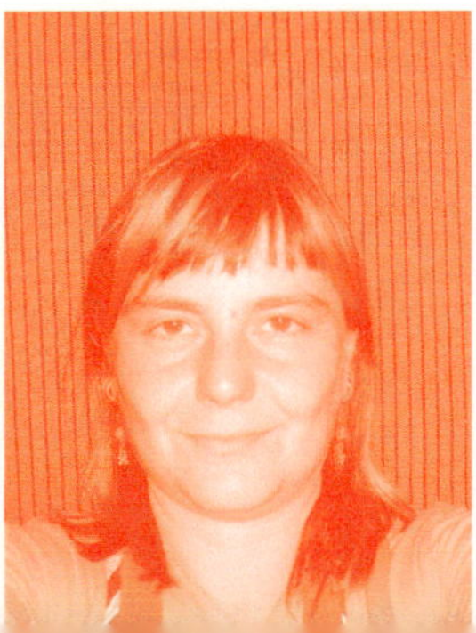

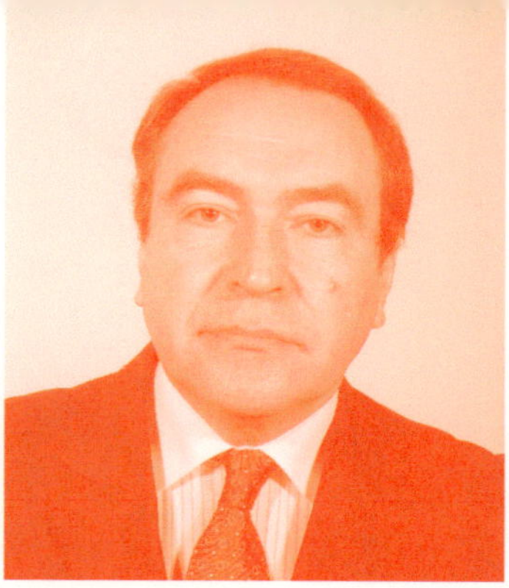
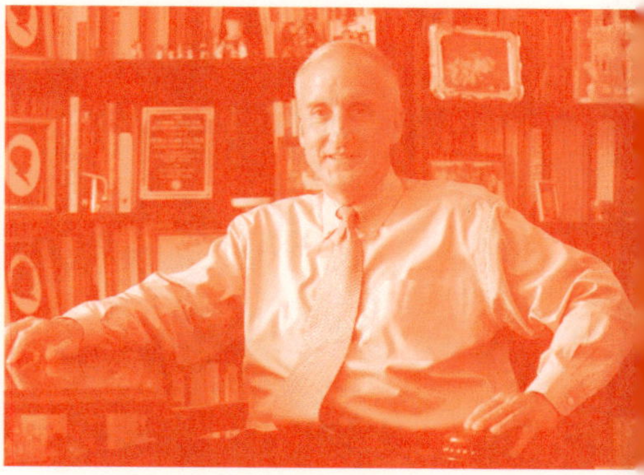
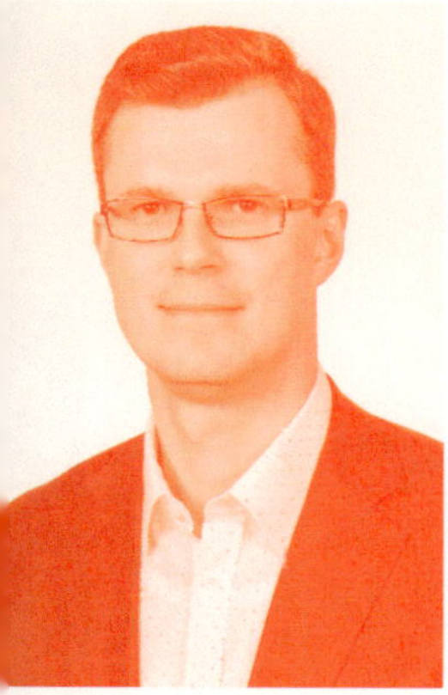
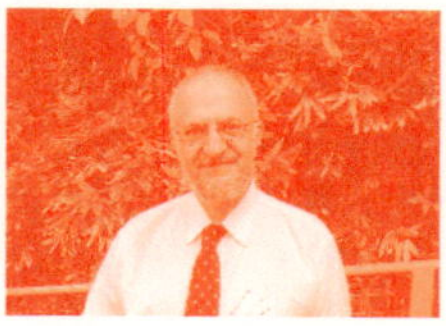
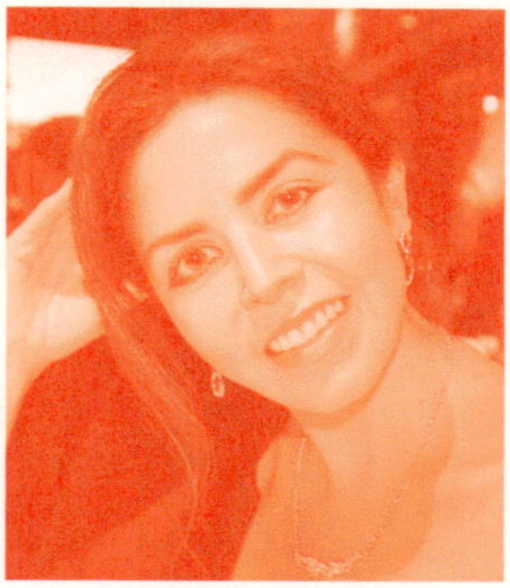

Supporting open minds since 2005

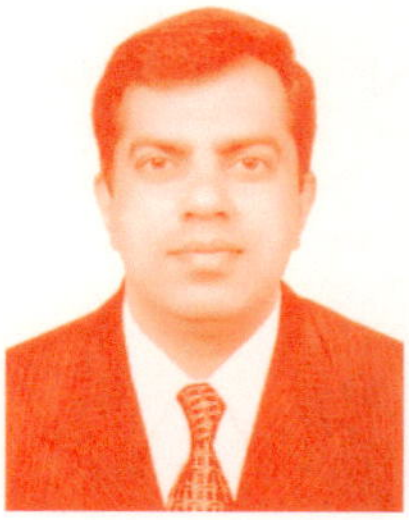
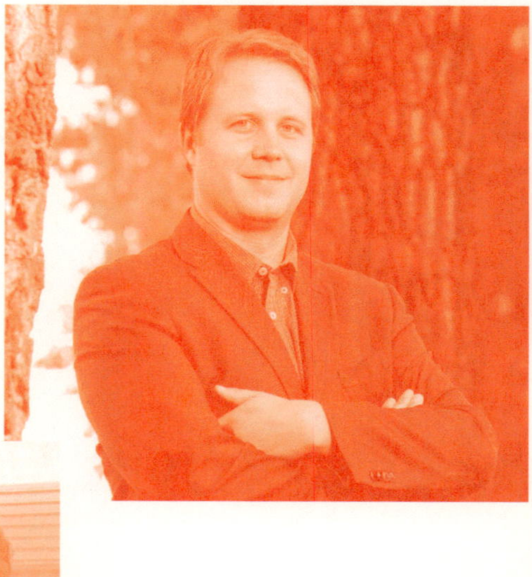
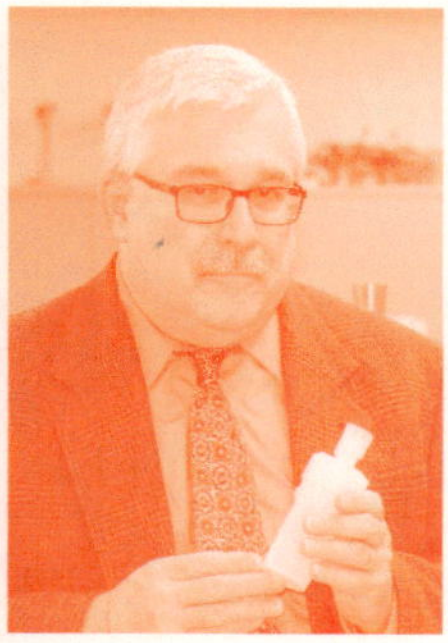
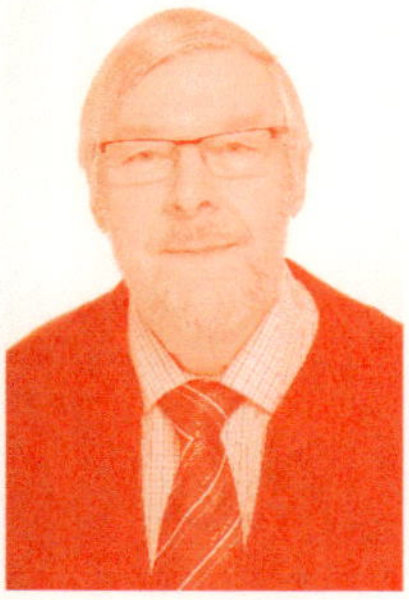
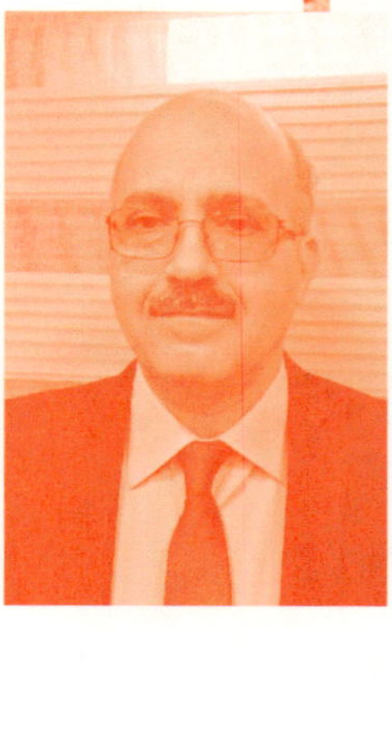
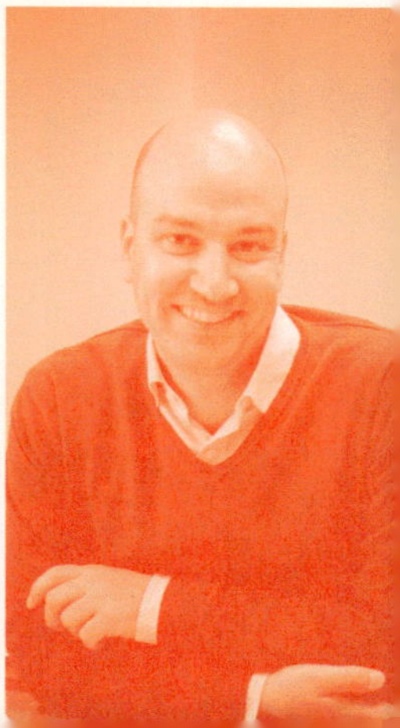
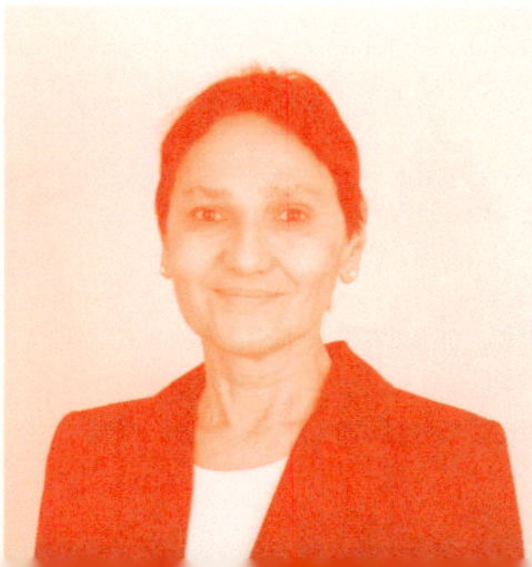

Recent Advances in Digital System Diagnosis and Management of Healthcare
http://dx.doi.org/10.5772/intechopen.83130
Edited by Kamran Sartipi and Thierry Edoh

Contributors
Joseph P. P. Lyons, Kimberly Watson, Angela Perez-Massacci, Norman Archer, Anait Gabrielyan, Mehrdad Roham, Kristen Miller, Robin Littlejohn, Christian Boxley, Ronald Romero Barrientos, Bernardo Canovas Segura, Antonio Morales, Manuel Campos, Jose M. Juarez, Francisco Palacios, Emmanuel Andrès, K.L. Choy, Valerie Tang, H.Y. Lam, G.T.S. Ho, Paul K.Y. Siu, Alessandro Taddei, Luciano Ciucci, Gianluca Rocchi, Fabrizio Conforti, Pierluigi Festa, Giuseppe Santoro, Thierry Edoh, Nathalie Jeandidier, Samy Talha, Abrar-Ahmad Zulfiqar, Laurent Meyer, Noel Lorenzo Villalba, Thibault Bahougne, Mohamed Hajjam, Amir Hajjam El Hassani

© The Editor(s) and the Author(s) 2021
The rights of the editor(s) and the author(s) have been asserted in accordance with the Copyright, Designs and Patents Act 1988. All rights to the book as a whole are reserved by INTECHOPEN LIMITED. The book as a whole (compilation) cannot be reproduced, distributed or used for commercial or non-commercial purposes without INTECHOPEN LIMITED's written permission. Enquiries concerning the use of the book should be directed to INTECHOPEN LIMITED rights and permissions department (permissions@intechopen.com).
Violations are liable to prosecution under the governing Copyright Law.

cc BY

Individual chapters of this publication are distributed under the terms of the Creative Commons Attribution 3.0 Unported License which permits commercial use, distribution and reproduction of the individual chapters, provided the original author(s) and source publication are appropriately acknowledged. If so indicated, certain images may not be included under the Creative Commons license. In such cases users will need to obtain permission from the license holder to reproduce the material. More details and guidelines concerning content reuse and adaptation can be found at http://www.intechopen.com/copyright-policy.html.

Notice
Statements and opinions expressed in the chapters are these of the individual contributors and not necessarily those of the editors or publisher. No responsibility is accepted for the accuracy of information contained in the published chapters. The publisher assumes no responsibility for any damage or injury to persons or property arising out of the use of any materials, instructions, methods or ideas contained in the book.

First published in London, United Kingdom, 2021 by IntechOpen
IntechOpen is the global imprint of INTECHOPEN LIMITED, registered in England and Wales, registration number: 11086078, 5 Princes Gate Court, London, SW7 2QJ, United Kingdom
Printed in Croatia

British Library Cataloguing-in-Publication Data
A catalogue record for this book is available from the British Library

Additional hard and PDF copies can be obtained from orders@intechopen.com

Recent Advances in Digital System Diagnosis and Management of Healthcare
Edited by Kamran Sartipi and Thierry Edoh
p. cm.
Print ISBN 978-1-78985-881-5
Online ISBN 978-1-78985-882-2
eBook (PDF) ISBN 978-1-78985-604-0

For EU product safety concerns:
IN TECH d.o.o., Prolaz Marije Krucifikse Kozulić 3, 51000 Rijeka, Croatia, info@intechopen.com or visit our website at intechopen.com.

We are IntechOpen, the world's leading publisher of Open Access books

Built by scientists, for scientists

5,200+
Open access books available

127,000+
International authors and editors

150M+
Downloads

156
Countries delivered to

Our authors are among the
Top 1%
most cited scientists

12.2%
Contributors from top 500 universities

CLARIVATE ANALYTICS BOOK CITATION INDEX INDEXED

WEB OF SCIENCE™

Selection of our books indexed in the Book Citation Index
in Web of Science™ Core Collection (BKCI)

Interested in publishing with us?
Contact book.department@intechopen.com

Numbers displayed above are based on latest data collected.
For more information visit www.intechopen.com

Meet the editors

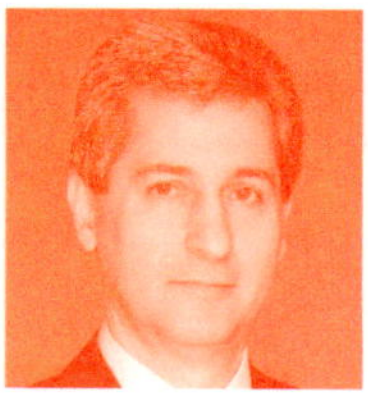

Dr. Kamran Sartipi is a faculty member in the Department of Computer Science at East Carolina University, Greenville, North Carolina, and an adjunct faculty member in the Information Systems at McMaster University, Ontario, Canada. Dr. Sartipi's education includes degrees in Electrical and Computer Engineering, and Computer Science and Software Engineering. His research activities are interdisciplinary including different aspects of intelligent decision systems through behavior pattern extraction, artificial intelligence, and big data analytics. Dr. Sartipi has long-term expertise in data analytics, knowledge engineering, intelligent decision systems, and software engineering, including successful applications in medical informatics and cybersecurity. He has more than eighty scientific publications in peer-reviewed journals and conferences. He has international research collaborations and trained several Ph.D. and master's students in interdisciplinary fields.

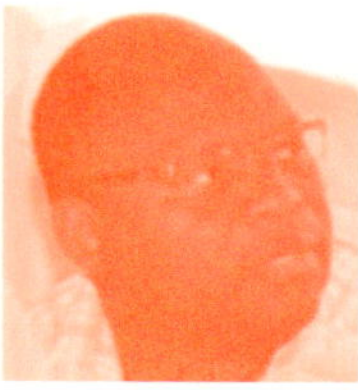

Thierry Oscar Edoh is an affiliated researcher at the University of Bonn, North Rhine-Westphalia, Germany (Drug Regulatory Affairs Program); visiting associate lecturer at the Institute of Mathematics and Physics (IMSP), University Abomey-Calavi, Benin, Africa; and visiting lecturer at the University Institute of Technology (IUT), Benin, Africa. Previously, he was an affiliated researcher in the Department of Applied Software Engineering at the Technical University of Munich, Germany. He received his diploma in Computer Sciences from the Technical University of Munich, Germany, and a Ph.D. in computer science from the German Federal Army University (Bundeswehr University), Munich, where he worked for several years on the improvement of rural health care provision and access to healthcare in developing countries using ITC systems. He has performed postdoctoral research works at the University of Bonn.

Contents

Preface

As the quality, applicability, and speed of digital systems in healthcare continue to increase, and as costs continue to decrease, a myriad of advances in healthcare applications continue to appear. The wide adoption of large and complex electronic health record (EHR) systems by healthcare institutions along with the vast amount of publicly available medical information through the Internet have significantly increased public expectations for higher quality healthcare. In addition, the overwhelming flow of information through a variety of sources causes distractions and challenging situations for care provisioning. Fortunately, recent advances in science and technology, high-performance computing platforms, and more attention to social aspects of computing can help the situation. This book addresses such issues through scientific and practical solutions and future research pathways.

The scope of digital systems in healthcare spans telemedicine, homecare provisioning, life-support systems, and public health management. The success of these systems is highly dependent on the targeted specialty, the systems' accuracy and usability, and quality of information. The use of proper information technology, user experience, computing power, and Internet access has been challenged in the design of such systems. Recently, the influence and success of machine learning science and technologies empowered by fast computing cores have provided new opportunities to develop decision systems that will improve usefulness through more adoption and retention.

This volume includes chapters that elaborate on the success of decision systems in different sectors of healthcare and medical domains and report on a number of these advances. In the first section on Digital Technology for Healthcare Management, Chapter 1 by Lyons et al. reports on the implementation of a national home telehealth program by the US Veterans Health Administration, noted for its advanced use of digital systems to support veterans. In Chapter 2, Andrès et al. provide a review of technologies and non-invasive devices for optimal management of diabetes mellitus, chronic heart failure, and related comorbidities. In Chapter 3, Edoh discusses primary healthcare service delivery and accessibility through digital technologies. Finally, in Chapter 4, Taddei et al. outline the telemedicine network for pediatric cardiology that is in use throughout thirteen hospitals located in the Tuscany region in Italy.

In the second section on Clinical Decision Support Systems (CDSS), Chapter 5 by Littlejohn et al. addresses the need to use human factors engineering to improve CDSS human interfaces. In Chapter 6, Siu et al. report on an intelligent CDSS that helps care managers to develop plans for better quality care in-home and institutional elderly care. In Chapter 7, Roham et al. present a systematic review of big data visualization to support more informative user interactions with CDSS. The section ends with Chapter 8 in which Segura et al. describe a system that supports gathering data from multiple sources on infections caused by resistant bacteria. Their system provides decision support to multi-institutional teams for fighting these threats.

Kamran Sartipi
East Carolina University,
USA

Thierry Edoh
University of Bonn,
Germany

Section 1

Digital Technology for Healthcare Management

Chapter 1

The Evolution of Elderly Telehealth and Health Informatics

Joseph P. Lyons, Kimberly Watson and Angela Massacci

Abstract

Many elderly individuals experience memory loss and often dementia as they age. This causes problems for the elderly due to diminished skills and increase in medical problems and natural decline. The Veterans Health Administration (VHA) introduced a national home telehealth program, Care Coordination/Home Telehealth (CCHT). Its purpose was to coordinate the care of veteran patients with chronic conditions and avoid their unnecessary admission to long-term institutional care. Such programs are cost-effective. Long-term care insurance companies are likely to cover these services. Home care and nursing home corporations are following the VHA's lead. We have recently witnessed significant advances in technology. Internet and mobile applications have opened a new world, providing information and opportunities for individuals to learn more information about illness and at a much faster rate. Smart home technology has evolved. Elderly patients often encounter difficulties using these technologies. Despite the advances in telehealth and telemedicine and the evolution of the technology, many individuals cannot afford the treatment or the technology. These same individuals and families are part of the digital divide, and they have not embraced the new technology. Federal programs have been developed and implemented to help this portion of the population.

Keywords: National Home Telehealth Program, Internet applications, Smart Home Technology, Telemedicine, Health Informatics

1. Introduction

As individuals age in the United States society, they receive benefits once they reach 65 years of age. They are considered senior citizens and receive many discounts from corporations as well as Social Security and Medicare financial benefits. The older individual frequently slows down mentally and physically. Many elderly individuals experience memory loss and often dementia as they age. This causes problems for the elderly due to diminished skills and increased medical problems and natural decline.

In the last 20 years, we have witnessed significant advances in technology. Internet and mobile applications have opened a new world, providing information and opportunities for individuals to learn more information about illness and at a much faster rate. Elderly patients often encounter difficulties using these technologies. Younger people adopt new technologies much easier, with much shorter learning curves. Internet and mobile applications are written by younger people and are more frequently used by them. The applications are not rewritten to make it easier for elderly people to use. Every day the elderly person encounters new problems such as physical ailments. The provost at a large public university stated "Every day I find a new problem or disability that I will have for the rest of my life" [1]. The technologies to resolve these problems are written by younger people who have many applications on their phones. The elderly person often does not have the interest to install these applications on his or her phone or to use the application. The elderly view such technologies as challenges rather than the benefits that they are designed to produce.

In this paper, we will examine how the elderly will adopt health information technology and the barriers to such adoption. We will then discuss the emergence of smart home technology and how it will be implemented in the homes of older adults. We will explore how caregivers will be trained and the impact of such training on the adoption of telehealth technology by the elderly. The groundbreaking work of the Veteran Administration with their introduction of Care Coordination/Home Telehealth (CCHT) will be discussed in detail. The hospital at home model introduced by Johns Hopkins University Hospitals will be explained. The evolution in health informatics and telehealth will also occur in nursing home corporations and home care companies. The rationale for such expansion will be explored. Recent technology advances in smart homes will be further discussed. The authors will then describe how an elderly person should go about implementing telehealth technology in his or her home and the efforts of academic institutions to develop training programs for caregivers and home care professionals.

2. Challenges to health information technology (HIT) adoption by older adults

Advances are being made in the implementation of the electronic health record (EHR), speech recognition, and telemonitoring with elderly patients in their homes. The electronic health record helps the elderly person keep track of their healthcare problems, such as which problem was treated by which health professional, when treatment occurred, and the outcome of those treatments.

EPIC software, a major electronic health record vendor in the United States, produces *MyChart* patient portal for all its patients and educates them on its use while in the hospital [2]. EPIC is the EHR system for many large healthcare organizations such as Cleveland Clinic, Geisinger Health System, and the Mayo Clinic. Other software vendors offer similar EHR chart products. Every year the elderly person will have outpatient visits to many different professionals, primary care, cardiologists, dentists, physical therapists, chiropractors, podiatrists, etc. Although each of these professionals has their own specialized EHR systems, the different vendors are building links to allow the systems to transfer information between different EHR systems. This is termed *interoperability*. The US federal government is constantly helping EHR vendors to make their systems communicate in a streamlined fashion. Fast Healthcare Interoperability Resources (FHIR) [3] is a standard to help achieve healthcare information systems' interoperability. FHIR uses HL7 messaging standards which are widely implemented by the healthcare industry and have been deployed internationally for decades. HL7 Version 2 health information exchange standards are a popular choice of local hospital communities for the exchange of healthcare information, including electronic medical record information [3].

Today's healthcare providers have a primary focus of improving elderly patient outcomes. Each healthcare facility faces a need to choose strategies that are most suitable to ensure provision of information system and communication technology

[4]. One of the key priorities for governments and healthcare providers around the world is postponing disability and dependency in later life [5]. Hospital-based patient portals have the potential to better inform and engage elderly patients in their care. MyChart is an electronic healthcare record portal that allows elderly patients online access to their medical records. These records are secured to provide privacy for the elderly patient. Bedside mobile tablets are now available to elderly patients while they are inpatients. These tablets allow real-time views of their results. It also has the capability of communicating with the nursing staff via electronics. These coordinated care networks are designed to drive higher-quality care as well as give the elderly patient a sense of control over their healthcare.

Healthcare is now being aimed toward focusing on meaningful use of care by engaging the elderly patient through online access and bedside tablets, allowing coordination of their own care. This focus is directly related to future impact of such involvement with the patient knowledge, elderly patient knowledge, and how such engagement will affect the delivery of care. Lack of communication often leaves the elderly patients unclear as to why tests are being ordered and why specialists have been consulted; such tools will allow the open forum for real-time questions to be asked. The purpose of these tools is to resolve communication gaps between the healthcare team and the elderly patients. The term e-patient was coined long before the advent of Internet to describe patients who take an active role in their health and healthcare by being equipped, enabled, empowered, and engaged [6]. Although e-patient is a pioneering concept, this concept will be explored through transformational and innovative methodology of healthcare technology.

Communication and compliance have long been challenges to the healthcare system especially with the elderly demographics. Maintaining a comprehensive continuity of care between providers and elderly patients has been an important challenge to hospital settings and the healthcare teams. Elderly patients today are more complex than ever for a multitude of reasons. These elderly patient populations often have multiple active disease processes, undergo numerous tests, and receive complex treatments during any hospital stay. This complexity has been found to have incomplete comprehensive care and less optimal engagement in their care [7].

Electronic healthcare systems have changed and continue to evolve in all aspects of healthcare and the delivery of our care. As with any change, this initiative has caused excessive excitement, anxiety, resistance, and conflict in every aspect of the healthcare setting especially with the elderly. To successfully implement, manage, and lead toward use of electronic healthcare records, leadership must work directly with the clinical, administrative, and technical people in their organization along with special training to teach the elderly generation how to utilize this technology. Nursing theories provide a foundation for supporting and managing the enormous degree of change experienced by the healthcare system and the people within any healthcare system [6]. Currently there is no single comprehensive, generally accepted theoretical, or conceptual model of health or nursing informatics [6]. Some of the key components in theory-based learning principles can apply to both the healthcare team and the elderly patient-centered care. Each learner is an individual with their own approach to learning, meaningful information to support retention; active engagement and participation also support long-term retention; conceptual learning is enhanced with concrete realistic examples; learning is enhanced when the teaching includes cognitive, affective, and psychomotor domains in concert; and learning is contagious. These are all examples of theory-based learning for both healthcare and elderly patients [6]. Educators need to be cognizant of their patient population to utilize the age-appropriate approach when teaching the elderly patient.

Many hospitals have incorporated the education and teaching of the use of MyChart into their discharge process. After visit processes are no longer just an act of handing the patient a discharge paper to sign, which are strategic and purposeful. This is especially important for the elderly patient population. Most organizational healthcare teams have daily patient flow rounds. These rounds are designed to establish needs of the patients to include reporting of which patients have signed up for the use of MyChart. The discharge process has the independent codes for the patients printed on the discharge papers. The nurse spends time educating and teaching the elderly patient population how to sign up for the use of MyChart. Once these patients are signed up, they continue to teach them how to set up their post-discharge appointments with their healthcare teams. They are shown how to look up results from laboratory work, the reconciled medication list, future appointments, future screening testing that is necessary, and any essential needs that may be pertinent to the elderly patient. The nursing staff is trained to assess the cognitive level of comprehension of their patient in their teaching. The nurse must determine if the patient understands or needs reinforcement. This piece of education is integrated into the patient's permanent charting. Often the elderly patient has a caregiver of some sort accompanied with them to support the teaching of this elderly patient population. This is very important during the educational discharge process of the elderly. The entire process is a patient-centered care coordination related to the elderly patient population. This training on bedside tablets by the staff member occurs when the patients are in the hospital. This knowledge of how to use the technology can be more easily transferred to the patient in his or her home once the patient is discharged.

The use of MyChart and/or any other EHR is considered one of healthcare's performance measures. The key performance indicator (KPI) report is printed out monthly to give a score card for the performance measures. This metric is a well-defined performance measurement used to monitor, analyze, and optimize healthcare processes to increase patient satisfaction and patient quality care. The use of this score card is to determine if the organization is meeting targets that are set up for the EHR in the system. These reports give a scorecard of the activation rate and percentage, the patient satisfaction rate with the access, and the domestic utilization related to the use of MyChart or electronic information technology. There is no data to determine age demographic yet with the KPI scorecard.

Another modality linked to the MyChart capability is the MyChart Evisit. An Evisit is an online visit available through MyChart with a primary care provider. This is a fast, affordable, and secure way to receive an online diagnosis and treatment plan for common medical conditions. It allows the elderly patient to remain in their home and still manage their healthcare needs. All communication related to the Evisit occurs in writing. There is no video, visual, photo, or verbal contact between the elderly patient and the primary care provider. This modality allows the elderly patient to seek medical advice for low acuity conditions. The patient fills out an available questionnaire about their symptoms and submits to a provider. There is a general charge of $36 for the Evisit. Many insurance plans cover the Evisit; however, the coverage does vary. The Evisit is designed for nonurgent conditions. If the provider feels the condition requires an emergency room visit or in-person visit, they will cancel the Evisit and notify the patient via online MyChart.

Here are some of the common conditions that are available for an Evisit:

Acute eVisits	Chronic condition follow-up eVisits
Sinus, cold, and/or cough	Seasonal allergies follow-up
Back pain	Insomnia follow-up

Acute eVisits	Chronic condition follow-up eVisits
Diarrhea	Hypothyroid follow-up
Urinary problems	Hypertension follow-up
Heartburn	IBS follow-up
Headache	Osteoarthritis follow-up
Rash	Diabetes follow-up
Vaginal discharge	Migraine follow-up
Pink eye	

The direct patient access via patient portal, MyChart, is designed to improve patient engagement with the elderly population. It is believed that through this access the elderly patients will feel a sense of ownership of their results and patient care. The ability to view results is another modality available through MyChart for the elderly patient population. It is thought that if elderly patients can view results prior to visiting their physicians, it would allow time to absorb and prepare with valid questions regarding their healthcare. One goal that is noted is that making abnormal test results available to the elderly patient population would improve patient safety by increasing the likelihood of elderly patients following up on the abnormal results [8]. This is believed to increase compliance with this elderly patient population which will have a direct impact on nursing and patient care. The approach of delivering the patient portal direct access is to manage the process that may result in more effective and efficient healthcare delivery system [6]. This technology described is to assist in nursing practice to accommodate in education and teaching methods for the elderly patients. This education and teaching is designed to directly impact the patient care for the aging patient population through increased compliance and knowledge regarding their medical condition.

When dealing with any healthcare records, there is always the ethical consideration to be considered. Electronic medical records are beneficial in a multitude of ways; however, security and confidentiality are of upmost importance regarding the data. The patient has the right to have their information. This information is only to be released to unauthorized persons with the consent of the individual. Of course, there must be consensual documentation for participants to be included in any kind of research or study performed. Data integrity refers to the accuracy and consistency of stored and transmitted data that can be compromised when information is entered incorrectly or deliberately altered [6]. Privacy and confidentiality are at the forefront of concerns when it comes to electronic healthcare records. Despite regulatory requirements and governed control of records, major issues related to privacy and security need to be addressed prior to nationwide interoperable EHR being fully implemented [6]. Patient portals will be secured by security and pass codes that only patients will have access to. There is the thought that the elderly patient population will be apprehensive about the fact that if they can have mobile access to their information, so may the public. This apprehension related to privacy of healthcare information is one of the challenges that healthcare providers need to be forthright about when dealing with the elderly patient population. There is still the ambivalence of protection of information with the elderly. Despite this barrier, healthcare providers maintain the initiative to educate and bring the elderly on board with new technology and the benefits to this patient population.

Some elderly patients use healthcare standard systems like Microsoft HealthVault since it provides a platform in which the individual can merge their healthcare information [9]. The purpose of electronic health records is to provide a vehicle where all the patient's records can be stored. Each of his or her providers can identify all the treatments and results that the patient has received. Since interoperability between such EHR systems has not been achieved, the patient often turns to HealthVault to combine all his or her records. Since the elderly person visits many providers, he/she or a family member can use HealthVault to merge their EHR records. Health information technology programs are written and used by young people. The elderly use technology less frequently and are not as familiar with the options and health information technology processes. In addition to electronic health records, the elderly will need to learn several pieces of this new health technology. Elderly who have used computers in their recent work life are more likely use HIT in retirement [10]. Lack of trust in HIT systems is often a major barrier. Numerous passwords and unfamiliar HIT procedures may also cause problems for the elderly and reduce usage.

For 60 years, the elderly population has relied on professionals for healthcare. Elders were asked to rank information received according to their level of trust. Health information on the Internet ranked behind clinical HIT sources and magazines and newspapers [11]. Elders are vulnerable to scams and abuse, especially with financial and healthcare and prescription drugs [12]. Wild et al. [13] found that older adults in home settings will accept surveillance and sharing of health information if it can be used by their physicians to preserve the elderly person's health. The network of sensors monitors the condition of the subject under supervision and sends the information to a distant healthcare facility over the Internet [14], or it can automatically call for EMS in case of an emergency. Some physicians are strongly encouraging their staff members to take the time to help the elderly person learn how to access health information data and use telehealth and telemedicine technology. Many organizations and practices offer additional training for staff members related to HIT but are especially aimed toward providing the necessary tools to educate the elderly population.

Interoperability among different treatment protocols and standards is also critical for the consistent operation of the system. In addition, precise and accurate measurements of key health parameters are vital for a reliable health monitoring system. The advancement of miniaturized and inexpensive sensors, embedded computing devices, and wireless networking technologies is paving the way for the utilization of remote health monitoring systems. Remote health monitoring allows unobtrusive, ubiquitous, and real-time monitoring of physiological signs without interrupting the daily activities of individuals.

Patients are now able to remain in their familiar home environment and enjoy their normal lives with friends and family while their health is being monitored and analyzed from a remote facility based on the physiological data collected by different on-body sensors. The system can perform a long-term health trend analysis, detect anomalies, and generate alert signals in case of an emergency. The problem may be that the elderly person must remove these sensors to complete some activities of daily living such as showering or bathing and then may forget to put the sensors back on. This is a burden that each elderly person who has sleep apnea experiences each evening even though the technology has been in place for several years and the sleep apnea process is well known to the elderly person.

By most estimates, the average trip to the emergency room (ER) in the USA costs $1500 to $2500. Recent research from the Centers for Disease Control estimated the number of trips per year to be 136.3 million [15]. The CDC's research also showed that the number of injury-related visits to the ER was 40.2 million, meaning that the other nearly 100 million visits might have been avoided with preventative care. A visit to a doctor's office costs significantly less on average than a trip to the ER, so the USA and other countries are desperately trying to find a way to cut down on the number of avoidable ER trips made each year. The cost of such visits can be further reduced using telemedicine and telehealth.

3. The emergence of smart home technology

"One of the possible solutions is the development of smart medical homes that can measure patient health and alert both the individual and a medical professional if a problem arises. These homes—and the individuals themselves—can be outfitted with machine-to-machine (M2M) medical devices that use sensors to monitor patient health and can transmit information to healthcare workers. So, what would a smart medical home look like? One feature might be to have the individual connected to a wearable device that monitors glucose levels for a diabetic patient. Even the person's sneakers could be outfitted with sensors that function as gait monitors to measure changes in walking patterns, stumbling and falling. Over time such devices would detect a limp or shuffle that could be a symptom of a more serious illness or injury. As these kinds of products become staples of the home environment, they will occupy a larger piece of the total M2M market. Recent market analysis from Juniper Research, for example, projects the smart wireless healthcare and fitness device services market will reach $1.8 billion by 2019" [16]. Because home-based M2M medical devices monitor critical vital signs, they must be supported by reliable wireless connectivity and have the capacity to transmit data steadily and quickly.

"Long-Term Evolution (LTE) has been recently introduced. Because LTE is a cellular connection rather than Wi-Fi, a patient can be monitored anywhere there is LTE coverage" [17]. This flexibility allows them to enjoy their independence without worrying about staying connected. A 4G LTE certainly fits the bill, but for many years the technology was considered too expensive and consumed too much power to be viable for these kinds of devices. That paradigm is now shifting, with the advent of low-power 4G LTE chipsets that conserve power and battery life by controlling data flow. These chipsets make the prospect of building 4G capability into devices more financially feasible for manufacturers and will, ultimately, increase adoption of connected medical technology. On top of the potentially massive economic benefits these new-age homes may provide, they will also help at-risk individuals avoid medical scares and give their families peace of mind. In other words, the smart medical home concept is moving forward and 4G LTE will help push it along. For this technology to be implemented, the elderly person will have to embrace this technology. Herein lies the problem, the elderly person will have to learn how to implement the technology and how to use it effectively. Caregivers will need to be trained so that he or she can help the elderly learn about the technology, implement it, and use the technology on a daily basis. For example, sleep apnea technology is used effectively by the elderly population on a daily basis.

4. Caregivers help the elderly

Numerous Internet and mobile applications have been recently developed which target caregivers for care coordination [18]. If the patient suffers from dementia, there are tools which focus on improving caregiver's ability to help the person to reduce their care burden [19]. The needs of the caregivers are quite different than those of the elderly. The caregiver may be better able to use the technology than the elderly client. The elderly client may be able to be taught how to use the HIT by the caregiver. This will depend on the training program available to the caregiver and the elderly person. As HIT expands, such teaching may grow into a large part of the caregiver's work in the near future. Teaching the elderly person to use the Internet for health information resulted in the elderly being willing to use the Internet more often [20]. Barriers to decision-making using HIT, information, and communication issues are modifiable [21]. Technology may be the means for the elderly to overcome those barriers [22]. The authors of this paper envision the emergence of laboratories at universities and private business where these skills are taught and certification courses are offered. Home care companies and nursing home corporations will more than likely lead the way and help train the caregivers as well as the elderly themselves. This training will also provide some burden relief of the caregivers and reduce caregiver burnout.

5. Veterans Health Administration (VHA) introduces Care Coordination/Home Telehealth

"Between July 2003 and December 2007, the Veterans Health Administration (VHA) introduced a national home telehealth program, Care Coordination/Home Telehealth (CCHT). Its purpose was to coordinate the care of veteran patients with chronic conditions and avoid their unnecessary admission to long-term institutional care. CCHT involves the systematic implementation of health informatics, home telehealth, and disease management technologies. It helps elderly patients live independently at home. CCHT is now a routine service provided by VHA to support veteran patients with chronic conditions as they age. CCHT patients are predominantly male (95%) and aged 65 years or older. The VHA uses strict criteria to determine patient eligibility for enrollment into the program. The VHA staff assesses how well its CCHT programs meet standardized clinical, technology, and managerial requirements" [23].

"The VHA trained 5000 staff to provide CCHT. Routine analysis of data obtained for quality and performance purposes from a cohort of 17,025 CCHT patients showed the benefits of a 25% reduction in numbers of bed days of care, 19% reduction in numbers of hospital admissions, and mean satisfaction score rating of 86% after enrollment into the program. The cost of CCHT was $1,600 per patient per annum, substantially less than other NIC programs and nursing home care" [23].

Here is the cost analysis of the expected benefit of the VHA CCHT program:

1. $225/day × 17,025 patients × 365 days = $13,981,781,000

2. 25% reduction = $10,486,335,000

3. Savings due to using CCHT = $3,495,446,000

4. Saving per patient $3,495,446,000/17025 patients = $20,531 per patient

The projected number of people over 65 in the USA is 46 million [24].

Let's be conservative and assume that 30% of the elderly (65+) are in need of treatment and can benefit from programs such as CCHT: The Veterans Health Administration estimates that 75,000, or about 50%, of its total patient population, could be cared for with home telemedicine technologies [23]. However in our analysis below, we will use 30%.

5. 46 million × .30 = 13.8 million people.

6. Savings from treating these 13.8 million people using CCHT is 13.8 × $20,531 = $2,833,278,000.

7. Estimates of CCHT savings = $2.833 billion.

The detailed reader may quarrel with the numbers, but it is evident that significant savings can be gained by implementing CCHT.

The VHA's experience is that an enterprise-wide home telehealth implementation is an appropriate and cost-effective way of managing chronic care patients in both urban and rural settings. This positive experience has set the stage for other governmental agencies and private home care and institutional organizations to develop and implement similar services for the elderly. The question is what percentage of the elderly can be trained to use telehealth technology and remain in their residence? 50 or 30 or 10%?

For veterans who have a health problem like diabetes, chronic heart failure, chronic obstructive pulmonary disease (COPD), depression, or post-traumatic stress disorder, getting treatment can be complex and inconvenient. For some, especially older veterans, conditions like these can make it difficult for them to remain living independently in their own home and make it necessary for them to go into a nursing home where their symptoms and vital signs (pulse, weight, temperature, etc.) can be checked frequently. Having this information means providers and nurses can change medications or other treatments and prevent serious health problems from developing.

Now there are new technologies that make it possible to check on symptoms and measure vital signs in the home. Special devices (home telehealth technologies) can do this and are easy to use for some elders. Home Telehealth (HT) can connect a veteran to a VHA hospital from home using regular telephone lines, cellular modem (these act as doors for transmission of information), and cell phones (using an interactive voice response system).

The VHA has found that not every patient is suitable for this kind of care. VA patients must be evaluated and trained. But, for those that are suitable for this kind of care, Home Telehealth can help them to remain at home and live independently. The VHA is hiring staff nurses to be home telehealth specialists. The VHA has demonstrated that Home Telehealth can be a cost-effective alternative to full-time residence in a nursing home. The VHA has demonstrated this technology for veterans.

Private nursing home corporations are following the VHA's lead offering the same technology to nonveterans. Private patient home services are financed by many different methods: long-term care insurance, Medicaid for eligible patients, limited Medicare for short periods, and private pay.

Here is a statement from a popular long-term care insurance company policy:

> *"MedAmerica [25] will provide Daily Benefits at 100% of the actual charges incurred up to the Maximum Nursing home Benefit amount shown in your Schedule of Benefits for Qualified Long-Term Care Services provided by a Nursing Home while you are a resident.*
> *If you are Benefit Eligible, MedAmerica will provide Daily Benefits at 100% of the actual charges incurred up to the Maximum Assisted Living Facility Benefit amount shown in your Schedule of Benefits for Qualified Long-Term Care Services provided in an Assisted Living Facility.*

> *If you are Benefit Eligible, MedAmerica will provide Daily Benefits at 100% of the actual charges incurred up to the Maximum Home Health Care or Adult Day Care Benefit amount shown in your Schedule of Benefits for Qualified Long-Term Care Services provided in a Home Health Care or an Adult Day Care Facility that are:*
>
> 1. *Home Health Care or personal care attendant services including such things as: personal hygiene, performing Activities of Daily Living, managing medications and other related support services.*
>
> 2. *Adult day care*
>
> 3. *nursing services*
>
> 4. *Physical, occupational, respiratory and speech therapy*
>
> 5. *Homemaker services including light work, household tasks, preparing meals, doing laundry and other incidental household tasks that do not require the services of a trained aide or attendant."*

Although the authors of this paper are not lawyers, it appears to us that MedAmerica and other long-term care insurers will cover the cost of HIT and HT as well as assist the caregivers in the elder's home.

Several commercial vendors are offering similar telehealth products. Listed below are a few examples:

1. Live Expert is advertised as the "next-generation home healthcare system and remote patient monitoring" [26].

2. HoneyCo, based in Nashville, offers a one-stop shop for the smart home, taking products off the shelf and assembling them into a single, easy-to-use software-hardware platform [27].

As stated above, Home Telehealth technology provides a telemedicine tool for patients to take an active role in the management of their chronic diseases. HT works by allowing patients to transmit vital health data from their home to physicians' offices and, in turn, receive health coaching from their providers based on the clinical data they transmit. A home telehealth system generally consists of a standalone hub device that collects physiologic data from peripheral devices and connects the patient to the provider via interactive/audio/video capabilities. HT tools include audio and video conferencing capabilities, allowing remotely located healthcare professionals to interview, observe, and educate the patient. In addition, HT tools assist in the use of the peripherals or other medical devices. Once again most elderly individuals and couples will need assistance to implement and use this technology daily. The VHA has demonstrated that this can occur and is occurring for eligible and willing veterans. This telehealth technology is transferable to the general population.

Advanced HT tools have the ability to show full-motion video, which can be used to provide patient education. HT tools include audio and video conferencing capabilities, allowing remotely located healthcare professionals to interview, observe, and educate the patient. In addition, HT tools assist in the use of the peripherals or other medical devices.

Despite the large number of health information technologies available in the marketplace, the current installed base of devices still remains relatively small, particularly in light of the immense target population of chronically ill patients. The majority of devices currently in use are still part of pilot or demonstration projects [28].

6. VA expands telehealth services again with T-Mobile's 70,000 lines

1. *"The US Department of Veterans Affairs and T-Mobile announced that T-Mobile would be adding 70,000 lines of wireless service to increase telehealth services in the VA network and expand services to veterans, especially those in rural areas [29]. The expanding network will connect veterans at home and at VA facilities, such as community-based outpatient clinics (CBOCs), with VA clinicians within the VA network.*

2. *This adds to VA's push this year to extend telehealth to distant veterans in rural areas through initiatives such as with T-Mobile and the Spok Health – Standard Communications partnership to expand the Spok Care Connect messaging service to more VA healthcare systems. The VHA (Veterans Health Administration) has long been the largest user of telehealth services in the US. Until recently, their emphasis has been on store-and-forward and clinic-based patient consults, but finally Home Telehealth (HT) is being supported. Reportedly, only 1% of veterans used Home Telehealth, while 12% used other forms of telehealth. The VA was among the earliest users of remote patient monitoring/home telehealth, dating back to 2003 and even earlier, with companies such as Viterion and Cardiocom.*

3. *While most of the news about VA has been about their leadership changes and their difficulties around EHRs, their 'Anywhere to Anywhere' program was finalized in May 26, 2018. This allows VA practitioners to provide virtual care across state lines to veterans, regardless of local telehealth regulations.*

4. *T-Mobile is already the lead wireless provider to the VA. The 70 K line addition is part of the carrier's $993.5 million five year contract with the US Navy."* The impact of this telehealth expansion will not only facilitate the use by veterans but will lead the way for the private sector to implement telehealth, especially in rural areas.

7. The hospital at home model, Johns Hopkins University Schools of Medicine and Public Health

The VHA, along with other major hospital systems, is exploring methods to discharge patients and continue treatment in the patient's home. The following section depicts the work done at Johns Hopkins on the hospital at home project.

The *hospital at home model* was developed by the Johns Hopkins University Schools of Medicine and Public Health. The framework has been adopted by a number of hospitals around the country, including Veterans Affairs and integrated delivery systems with Medicare Advantage Plans. This model was designed to care for acutely ill patients within their homes. The primary target population is elderly patients with multiple chronic conditions and acute illness or those experiencing exacerbations of their chronic conditions and requiring acute hospital care. Treating patients in the home can save money, reduces the risk of health threats for the patients (especially for this at-risk population), and opens up hospital beds for other patients.

In 2012, the hospital at home program treated more than 1000 patients throughout the country. These patients are at low risk of clinical deterioration with proper care and are not likely to require highly technical, hospital-based procedures. Hopkins' initial research focused on frail, chronically ill, elderly patients who required acute hospital admission for one of the following reasons: (a) community-acquired pneumonia, (b) heart failure exacerbation, (c) chronic obstructive pulmonary disease exacerbation, and (d) Cellulitis Complex Care Management Program.

This program overview is part of a series describing innovative approaches to caring for complex patients. Funded by the California Health Care Foundation, these overviews are the result of a national scan highlighting programs active in the field that have demonstrated success. "*After their national demonstration study, Hopkins added several other conditions, including: Deep vein thrombosis (DVT); Pulmonary embolism (PE); Dehydration/volume depletion; and Complicated UTI/Urosepsis. The program does not include patients on dialysis. Patients do not have to have a caregiver. The process of patient identification differs among the adoption sites. Patients can be identified using electronic health records, physician referrals, or other methods, such as emergency department (ED) referral*" [30].

Johns Hopkins found that implementation of the program on a wide scale has been limited by the incorrect assumption that hospital care is safer and bypasses payment issues with Medicare. Currently, there are no payment codes for hospital at home care in fee-for-service Medicare. Thus, implementation of the hospital at home model has been limited to Medicare managed care, integrated delivery systems, and Veterans Affairs health systems. A challenge of the model is the difficulty in serving patients across a broad geography. Successful implementations of this model have limited the geography to a 20- or 30-mile radius from the hospital.

The VHA Clinical Research Study of 2007 [23] and the Johns Hopkins hospital at home model have more than adequately demonstrated that such elderly health informatics systems can be effective for at least 30% of the elderly population. We think the training of the patients in the hospitals and the caregivers along with having physician's staff support facilitating the efforts will be instrumental in the elderly embracing this technology. The elderly population are now much more inclined to own and use cell phones than in previous years. They use the Internet to bypass the cable companies and stream television programs on their 4K televisions. Consumer cellular and other phone companies have carved out a business by focusing on the elderly.

8. Nursing home corporations and home care companies

As technology evolves and becomes commonplace, will the large nursing home corporations such as Shepherd of the Valley, Ohio Living—Park Vista, Windsor House, Wesley Village, and Copeland Oaks Retirement Community—and several other corporations across the USA see this as competition? Or will they embrace this new technology and make HIT and HT part of their array of services? Will the home care companies see this as an opportunity to expand their healthcare role? The authors of this paper believe that both the nursing home companies and the home care companies will embrace this technology, lead the way, and offer these services to their clients. We expect that retirement communities will build telehealth technology into their single-family homes and the hospitals will also build such technology into the retirement apartments located adjacent to the hospitals. The evolution of this technology is just now starting to surface at a growing rate in the elderly population. It is believed as the upcoming years improve upon and master this technology that eventually it will become expected from all patient populations and especially the elderly.

9. The technology that will be functional in smart homes

"Smart homes, which incorporate environmental and wearable medical sensors, actuators, and modern communication and information technologies, can enable continuous and remote monitoring of elderly health and wellbeing at a low cost. Smart homes may allow the elderly to stay in their comfortable home environments instead of expensive and limited healthcare facilities. Healthcare personnel can also keep track of the overall health condition of the elderly in real-time and provide feedback and support from distant facilities" [31]. The elderly may require frequent, immediate medical intervention, which may otherwise result in fatal consequences. Such emergency situations can be avoided by monitoring the physiological parameters and activities of the elderly in a continuous fashion [32]. In most emergency cases, the elderly seek in-patient care, which is very expensive and can be a serious financial burden on the patient if the hospital stay is prolonged [33].

Remote health monitoring in a smart home platform, on the other hand, allows people to remain in their comfortable home environment rather than in expensive and limited nursing homes or hospitals, ensuring maximum independence to the occupants [34]. In recent years, the Internet of Things (IoT) has gained much attention from researchers, entrepreneurs, and tech giants [35] around the globe. The IoT is an emerging technology that connects a variety of everyday devices and systems such as sensors, actuators, appliances, computers, and cellular phones, thus leading toward a highly distributed intelligent system capable of communicating with other devices and human beings. The dramatic advancements in computing and communication technologies coupled with modern low-power, low-cost sensors, actuators, and electronic components have unlocked the door of ample opportunities for the IoT applications. The smart home with integrated e-health and assisted living technology is an example of an IoT application that can potentially play a pivotal role in revolutionizing the healthcare system for the elderly. The full details of this technology are beyond the scope of this paper, but the reader can find significant detail in the previously referenced sensors article [31].

Older adults with complex care needs want to live as independently as they can for as long as they can and limit stress on family and other caregivers. Telehealth strategies offer the potential to improve access to care and the quality of care while reducing strain on caregivers. For healthcare systems, home telehealth may help address the challenge of rising costs. Though limited today, home telehealth is likely to be implemented more widely as policy makers reduce regulatory barriers and providers focus on improving telehealth strategies to meet the needs of families.

The care of older adults with frailty, chronic disease, or significant disabilities who live in the community is a major challenge for both health systems and families [36]. This care can be sometimes rewarding yet simultaneously difficult for family caregivers to manage because of the lack of coordinated care and because of caregivers' competing obligations. As the nation ages, the number of frail older adults with functional and cognitive impairments who require assistance from others will increase. Consequently, planning for the care of people with complex chronic conditions has taken on greater urgency. Providing higher-quality and more cost-effective care for older adults with complex conditions will require models of care that, among other things, better integrate healthcare and social services and improve supports for family caregivers. To help achieve these goals, telehealth services are increasingly included as a component of community-based care for chronic conditions, mental health, and even palliative care. Through telehealth, providers can deliver a wide range of diagnostic, therapeutic, and care management services, as well as services to support caregivers, such as communication tools with clinicians, services that otherwise would be delivered in a healthcare setting or through in-person home visits. Telehealth has the potential to be an effective tool for improving access and continuity, improving outcomes, and lowering costs. Can the elderly population afford such expense? The answer is yes for a large percentage of the elderly. *Forbes* magazine [37] in March 2018 stated that elderly Americans in the 75+ age group had a mean net worth of $692,100. The typical net worth of the average retiree 65 years and older is $264,750.

The 2016 Federal Reserve Consumer Finance Survey purports there is a national shift toward wealth within the elderly population. There was an upward trend toward the incomes in those over age 75. The report also shows that the increase has occurred rapidly over a 30-year period. This leaves the senior population in the position to create financial support for their families. This fact has created a respect for America's elderly in their ability to support generations of children and grandchildren. The new reality for the elderly in Americans is that they are much more affluent than even those in their 50s. Comparing the data against that of the incomes of the 1950s, the wealth has reversed from the younger Americans to senior citizens [38]. The poverty level for seniors began improving in the 1960s and grew to be equal in wealth to other age groups by the 1980s.

10. Technology implementation is influenced by the "digital divide"

There are still some elderly that experience poverty [39, 40]. There are many that do not have access to the Internet and thus the many online services available for health prevention and promotion. There is some technological division that exists for the poor and rich. Those educated and higher-income seniors are significantly more inclined to have electronic and Internet resources to provide access to a large menu of software programs to manage health issues. There are many challenges in today's society for those who are not technologically skilled. There is a correlation between low income and low access to technology. There is also a direct link to the challenged socioeconomical population and increased physical impairments. This increase in patient impairments provides an even greater need to introduce this technology to such economically challenged elderly populations.

- According to the 2012 Pew Report "Digital Differences," only 62% of people in households making less than $30,000 a year used the Internet, while in those making $50,000–74,999, that percentage jumped to 90.

- Smartphones have helped bridge the divide, as they provide Internet access to populations previously at a digital disadvantage. Pew reports that, among smartphone owners, "young adults, minorities, those with no college experience, and those with lower household income levels" are more likely to access the Internet primarily through their phones.

- There are still gaps in high-speed Internet access. Only 49% of African Americans and 51% of Hispanics have high-speed Internet at home, as compared with 66% of Caucasians. Internet speed has important effects on media access, especially when it comes to streaming video, so this gap is significant.

A pilot program took place during the Obama Administration whereby the United States Department of Housing and Urban Development (HUD) worked with private businesses and nonprofit agencies to provide Internet assistance to low-income families. The ConnectHome Project brought light to the marked division in those who have easy access to Internet services and the income barrier that exists for many vulnerable groups, including the elderly. The pilot gave 38 communities the special Internet access services. There are many business and organizations that have expectations that the consumer has Internet access. This creates many access barriers for those who lack understanding or income to have Internet access.

The company Comcast has created an impact by providing low-cost Internet hardware and services. There have been over 2 million low-income Americans that have been assisted. The company has committed to offering training and support to assist with the Internet and computer literacy, making the technology purposeful for the people. The company identified any child in the school system who is eligible to receive free or reduced lunch would also determine that these families are qualified to get the assistance. The family will receive the service but also the broadband receiver. There are some that argue governmental involvement is crucial with the Internet divide. Without the support, there would be a larger division by blocking many Americans from educational or employment opportunities. The holistic approach to the problem seems to be creating a positive impact on the barriers that inhibit many from access. The question is Will AT & T, Spectrum, and other Internet providers provide specialized services to the elderly to facilitate the use of not only the Internet but also telehealth and health informatics technology?

11. Implementing telehealth technology in the patient's home

Telehealth and telemedicine are innovative technologies that deliver healthcare to the patient population. Telemedicine is the practice of medicine via technology to deliver healthcare at a distance. It enables the physician in one location using telecommunications infrastructure to deliver care to a patient at a distant site. Telehealth refers broadly to electronic and telecommunication technologies and services used to provide healthcare and services at a distance. The difference between the two is one where Telehealth refers to a broader scope of remote healthcare services than that of telemedicine.

Patients and caregivers have concerns related to the security, dependability of Internet connection, privacy protection, and how this assessment will be performed. These are all very valid concerns that have been addressed via secure and dependable Internet connection, custom-configured hardware and peripherals, custom software (electronic medical records (EMR)). One of the main vital must haves for Telehealth/Telemedicine is to secure an Internet connection. This is largely due to the involvement of consultations from a distance. Efforts are being made to build a stronger broadband infrastructure throughout the USA. The National Broadband Plan was initiated in 2010 by the US government to help ensure that all communities will have access to broadband service by 2020. "Broadband-enabled health information technology (IT) can improve care and lower costs by hundreds of billions of dollars in the future decades...." [41]. There have been billions of dollars in funding to support the National Broadband Plan by the congress. Healthcare providers are responsible for their own Internet connections.

There are technology grants available to some providers, especially those in rural and underprivileged areas.

> *"The University of Arkansas for Medical Sciences (UAMS) and the Arkansas e-Link team was awarded $102 million by the National Telecommunications Information Administration (NTA) in 2012. This was in alignment with supporting a statewide $128 million broadband infrastructure to serve community institutions across Arkansas. The Arkansas e-Link teams have installed and/or upgraded broadband, interactive video units and public access personal computers all over the state. There have been roughly 3900 community institutions, 61,000 businesses and has reached more than 185,000 underserved families impacted from the Arkansas e-Link infrastructure" [41].*

Patient privacy laws remain managed much in the same way they do with an in-person visit to a facility or provider in a face-to-face visit regarding telehealth/telemedicine. Prior to the initial clinical consultation, patients are educated and informed on how their data will be managed. They are asked to sign a consent form that explains the format for which information will be used and accessed.

The customized software is required to be encrypted, and the software must meet HIPAA Federal security standards and guidelines when using the telehealth/telemedicine hardware. Patients are educated and taught to use additional security efforts for any mobile devices that they should use such as phones and/or tables. These security efforts are mainly password security to their device and the ability to remotely disable mobile devices that are lost or stolen. The Health Insurance Portability and Accountability Act (HIPAA) was passed in the USA in 1996. The HIPAA is to protect a patient's right to privacy in both face-to-face visits and teleservice consultations. All healthcare providers are legally bound by this law.

Telehealth/Telemedicine consultation custom-configured hardware includes carts, desktop/laptop computers, and tablets. Carts are used for clinical and educational purposes and are typically portable systems. The clinical carts are utilized to deliver patient care. The educational carts are used for training, meetings, interviews, etc. Each of the carts is designed to be customized to meet whatever the specific needs and specialties may include. They include Codec which is used to encrypt the patient data. The carts also generally have a monitor, camera, keyboard, and remote control. They also have a PC to store patient information. This includes the capability to view live images as well as take pictures to store and forward to other healthcare professionals if care is needed to be delivered everywhere. The customization is available for all needs of any Telehealth/Telemedicine providers. They are designed to use tools, called peripherals, to assess patient needs. There are cameras available for visualization needs such as dermatology or radiology. Some other peripherals include items such as vital sign monitors, digital stethoscopes, probes, spirometers, etc. Most consultations are done via desktop computers or a laptop computer. HIPAA-compliant software must be used for encryption and privacy to install on all devices that are utilized for Telehealth/Telemedicine purposes. Usually when dealing with an acute situation or emergency, then tablets, such as iPads, are used in other healthcare areas. This mobile technology enables an immediate connection between the patient population and healthcare professional regardless of location. Tablets are also intermittently used to monitor conditions and consult with their healthcare team. The authors of this document envision a growth of technical specialists who will aid the elderly and train the caregivers in implementing and maintaining this technology in good working order.

Custom software (electronic medical records) is designed to deliver a digital patient record that is forwarded to other healthcare professionals and facilities.

Encrypted data is delivered to ensure security and privacy for the patient. There are several companies in the market that develop software to customize to meet the needs of the Telehealth/Telemedicine patient and providers.

Future technology is growing to the point of more mobile apps and self-monitoring devices that will feed information directly to a patient's digital record and automatic notifications to a healthcare team if issues develop. As Telehealth/Telemedicine services become more utilized and accepted, the technology will continue to develop to meet the needs of the patient and healthcare provider as well as cost-effectiveness.

12. Conclusion

The Veterans Health Administration in their national home telehealth program, Care Coordination/Home Telehealth demonstrated that the care of veteran patients with chronic conditions can be delivered in the patient's home. Up to 50% of the veterans can avoid their unnecessary admission to long-term institutional care. Such programs are cost-effective. Long-term care insurance companies are likely to cover these services. Home care and nursing home corporations are following the VHA's lead. Significant advances in the Internet and mobile and telehealth technology have opened a new world, providing information and opportunities for individuals to learn more information about illness and at a much faster rate. Smart home technology has evolved.

However, the elderly often encounter difficulties using these technologies. Caregiver training programs are evolving based on the VHS-CCHT model. Universities across the USA are working with home care and nursing home corporations, utilizing private as well as federal and foundation funding to develop telehealth training centers. The projected gain is that nonveterans will be able to achieve similar success rates as the veterans have and avoid their unnecessary admission to long-term institutional care.

Despite the advances in Telehealth and Telemedicine and the evolution of the technology, many individuals cannot afford the treatment or the technology. These same individuals and families are part of the digital divide, and they have not embraced the new technology. Federal programs have been developed and implemented to help this portion of the population. The learning curve of new technologies for the elderly population is changing. The knowledge gap will continue to close as the United States government supports more initiatives regarding health-related technology and its relationship to improved outcomes for the elderly.

Conflict of interest

The authors declare no conflict of interest.

Notes

The authors would like to recognize the authors of primary Ref. [42] because after reading this article, we were able to understand what was happening in the field of elder care and develop our own article.

Author details

Joseph P. Lyons[1*], Kimberly Watson[2] and Angela Massacci[2]

1 Youngstown State University, USA

2 Mercy Health, USA

*Address all correspondence to: jplyons@ysu.edu

IntechOpen

© 2020 The Author(s). Licensee IntechOpen. This chapter is distributed under the terms of the Creative Commons Attribution License (http://creativecommons.org/licenses/by/3.0), which permits unrestricted use, distribution, and reproduction in any medium, provided the original work is properly cited.

References

[1] Mosca J. Personal Communication. Interim Provost Youngstown State University; March 2019

[2] EPIC. Available from: https://www.epic.com/software

[3] FHIR: Fast Healthcare Interoperability Resources. Available from: http://hl7.org/implement/standards/fhir/ [20 Feb 2013]

[4] Potancok M, Vorisek J. Specific factors influencing information system/information and communication technology sourcing strategies in healthcare facilities. Health Informatics Journal. 2016;**22**:537-547. DOI: 10.1177/1460458215571644

[5] Witham MD, Frost H, McMurdo M, Donnan PT, McGilchrist. Construction of a linked health and social care database resource—Lessons on process, content and culture. Informatics for Health & Social Care. 2015;**40**:229-239. DOI: 10.3109/17538157.2014.892491

[6] Health Informatics: An Interprofessional Approach, 2nd ed. St. Louis, Missouri: Elsevier; 2018

[7] O'Leary KJ, Sharma RK, Killarney A, O'Hara LS, Lohman ME, Culver E, et al. Patients' and healthcare providers' perceptions of a mobile port application for hospitalized patients. BMC Medical Informatics and Decision Making. 2016: 1-8. DOI: 10.1186/s12911-016-0363-7

[8] Pillemer F, Price RA, Paone S, Martich GD, Albert S, Haidari MA. Direct release of test results to patients increases patient engagement and utilization of care. PLoS One. 2016;**11**: 1-9. DOI: 10.1371/journal.pone.0154743

[9] Microsoft HealthVault. Available from: https://www.healthvault.com/en-us/healthvault-for-consumers/

[10] Chun YJ, Patterson PE. A usability gap between older adults and younger adults on interface design of an Internet-based telemedicine system. Work. 2012;**41**(Suppl.1):349-352. DOI: 10.3233/wor-2012-0180-349

[11] Chaudhuri S, Le T, White C, Thompson H, Demiris G. Examining health information-seeking behaviors of older adults. Computers, Informatics, Nursing. 2013. DOI: 10.1097/01.NCN.0000432131.92020.42

[12] National Council on Aging (NCOA). Top 10 Scams Targeting Seniors. Washington, DC. 2013 [cited 2013 November 6]

[13] Wild K, Boise L, Lundell J, Foucek A. Unobtrusive in-home monitoring of cognitive and physical health: Reactions and perceptions of older adults. Journal of Applied Gerontology. 2008;**27**(2):181-200. DOI: 10.1177/0733464807311435 © 2008 The Southern Gerontological Society

[14] Talha U, Asif M, Mohan S, Ahmad J. Body area networks (BANs)—An overview with smart sensors based telemedical monitoring system. International Journal of Computer Applications. 2013;**84**(8)

[15] Jones S, Fox S. Generations Online in 2009. Pew Research Center; 2009. Available from: http://pewinternet.org/Reports/2009/Generations-Online-in-2009.aspx [Accessed: 28.01.09]

[16] Zickuhr K. Generations 2010. Pew Research Center; 2010. Available from: http://pewinternet.org/Reports/2010/Generations-2010.aspx [Accessed: 1]

[17] Vasavi B, Marepalli M, Gudur L. Evolution of 4G-research directions towards fourth generation wireless communication. International Journal of

Computer Science and Information Technologies. 2011;**2**(3):1087-1095

[18] The Regents of the University of California. PREPARE: Prepare for Your Care 2013. 2013. Available from: http://www.prepareforyourcare.org/ [cited 09.03.14]

[19] Topo P. Technology studies to meet the needs of people with dementia and their caregivers. A literature review. Journal of Applied Gerontology. 2009; **28**(1):5-37

[20] Campbell RJ, Nolfi DA. Teaching elderly adults to use the Internet to access health care information: Before-after study. Journal of Medical Internet Research. 2005;**7**(2):e19. DOI: 10.2196/jmir.7.2.e19 Epub 2005/07/07

[21] Bynum JP, Barre L, Reed C, Passow H. Participation of very old adults in health care decisions. Medical Decision Making. 2013. DOI: 10.1177/0272989X13508008

[22] Xie B, Wang M, Feldman R, Zhou L. Internet use frequency and patient-centered care: Measuring patient preferences for participation using the health information wants questionnaire. Journal of Medical Internet Research. 2013;**15**(7):e132. DOI: 10.2196/jmir.2615

[23] Darkins A, Ryan P, Kobb R, Foster L, Edmonson E, Wakefield B, et al. Care Coordination/Home Telehealth: The systematic implementation of health informatics, home telehealth, and disease management to support the care of veteran patients with chronic conditions. Telemedicine Journal and E-Health. 2008 Dec;**14**(10):1118-1126. DOI: 10.1089/tmj.2008.0021

[24] Colby SL, Ortman JM. Projections of the size and composition of the US population: 2014–2060: Population Estimates and Projections. 2017. Available from: wedocs.unep.org

[25] Lyons CJ. Personal communication. MEDIAMERICA'S POLICY STATEMENT Policy; 2014

[26] Live Expert list in search engines as "Next Generation Home Healthcare System & Remote Patient Monitoring"

[27] HoneyCo, based in Nashville, offers a one-stop shop for the smart home, taking products off the shelf and assembling them into a single, easy-to-use software-hardware platform

[28] Darkins A. The growth of telehealth services in the Veterans Health Administration between 1994 and 2014: A study in the diffusion of innovation. Telemedicine and e-Health. 2014. Available from: liebertpub.com

[29] Cusano D. VA Expands Telehealth Services Again with T-Mobile's 70,000 lines (26). Business Wire, Mobihealthne ws; December 13, 2018

[30] Cryer L, Shannon SB, Van Amsterdam M, Leff B. Costs For 'Hospital At Home' Patients Were 19 Percent—Health Affairs. Available from: https://www.healthaffairs.org/doi/pdf/10.1377/hlthaff.2011.1132

[31] Majumder S, Aghayi E, Noferesti M, Memarzadeh-Tehran H, Mondal T, Pang Z, et al. Smart homes for elderly healthcare—Recent advances and research challenges. Sensors. 2017; **17**(11):2496. DOI: 10.3390/s17112496

[32] Majumder S, Mondal T, Deen MJ. Wearable sensors for remote health monitoring. Sensors. 2017

[33] Torrance AD, Powell SL, Griffiths EA. Emergency surgery in the elderly: Challenges and solutions. Open Access Emergency Medicine. 2015;7: 55-68. DOI: 10.2147/OAEM.S68324. eCollection 2015

[34] Pantelopoulos A, Bourbakis N. A survey on wearable sensor-based

systems for health monitoring and prognosis. IEEE Transactions on Systems, Man, and Cybernetics: Part C Applications and Reviews. 2010

[35] Atzori L, Iera A, Morabito G. The internet of things: A survey. Computer Networks. 2010;**54**:2787-2805

[36] Quinn WV, O'Brien E, Spring G, Niehoff M. Using Telehealth to Improve Home-Based Care for Older Adults and Family Caregivers. May 14, 2018

[37] Howe N. The Graying Of Wealth. FORBES; March 16, 2018

[38] Flynn KE, Smith MA, Freese J. When do older adults turn to the internet for health information? Findings from the Wisconsin Longitudinal Study. Journal of General Internal Medicine. 2006;**21**(12): 1295-1301. DOI: 10.1111/j.1525-1497.2006.00622.x

[39] Digital Divide: The Technology Gap between the Rich and Poor. Available from: http://www.digitalresponsibility.org/digital-divide-the-technology-gap-between-rich-and-poor

[40] Roslyn M. Brock is the Chairman of the National Board of Directors for the NAACP. Who's poor in America? 50 years into the 'War on Poverty,' a data portrait https://www.pewresearch.org/fact-tank/2014/01/13/whos-poor-in-america-50-years-into-the-war-on-poverty-a-data-portrait/

[41] Lamp K. 3 Essential Technology Tools for use in Telehealth. Clinical, General, Growing Your Program, Technology, South Central Telehealth Resource Center, University of Arkansas for Medical Sciences; August 28th, 2015

[42] Fisher SH, David D, Crotty BH, Dierks M, Safran C. Acceptance and use of health information technology by community dwelling elders. International Journal of Informatics. 2014;**83**:624-625

Chapter 2

Actual as well as Future Technologies and Noninvasive Devices for Optimal Management of Diabetes Mellitus and Chronic Heart Failure

Emmanuel Andrès, Nathalie Jeandidier, Samy Talha, Abrar-Ahmad Zulfiqar, Laurent Meyer, Noel Lorenzo Villalba, Thibault Bahougne, Mohamed Hajjam and Amir Hajjam El Hassani

Abstract

In recent years, several technological innovations have become part of the daily lives of patients suffered from chronic diseases. It is the case for diabetes mellitus and chronic heart failure with noninvasive glucose sensors, intelligent insulin pumps, artificial pancreas, telemedicine, and artificial intelligence for an optimal management. A review of the literature dedicated to these technologies and devices supports the efficacy of the latter. Mainly, these technologies have shown a beneficial effect on diabetes or chronic heart failure management with mainly improvement for these two diseases of patient ownership of the disease; patient adherence to therapeutic and hygiene-dietary measures; the management of comorbidities (hypertension, weight, dyslipidemia); and at least, good patient receptivity and accountability. Especially, the emergence of these technologies in the daily lives of these patients suffered from chronic disease has led to an improvement of the quality of life for patients. Nevertheless, the magnitude of its effects remains to date debatable or to be consolidated, especially with the variation in patients' characteristics and methods of experimentation and in terms of medical and economic objectives.

Keywords: chronic disease, diabetes mellitus, chronic heart failure, noninvasive device, glucose sensors, intelligent insulin pumps, artificial pancreas, telemedicine, telemonitoring, artificial intelligence, Big Data

1. Introduction

According to the World Health Organization (WHO), "chronic disease" is defined as a long-term condition that changes over time, for example, high blood pressure, diabetes mellitus, chronic heart failure (CHF) or chronic obstructive

IntechOpen

pulmonary disorders (COPD), cancer, chronic kidney diseases, cognitive impairment and deterioration, etc. [1, 2].

In France, it is estimated that 15 million people (about 20% of the population) are projected to suffer from chronic disease compared to 30% of the population in Canada and in other developed countries [2].

To date, despite major therapeutic advances, most chronic diseases remain serious in terms of functional or survival prognosis, with high morbidity and mortality rates [1]. Yet, this type of disease is responsible for 17 million deaths worldwide each year. A 5-year mortality rate of 30–50% has been reported in patients with New York Heart Association (NYHA) stages III–IV CHF [3]. In this setting, patients also frequently present for emergency hospitalization and rehospitalization, with long hospital stays, resulting in impaired quality of life [1, 3]. In France, acute and chronic HF is thus responsible for over 210,000 hospitalizations per year [1, 2], accounting for 5% of all hospitalizations and being the main cause of hospitalization among elderly subjects.

Optimal management of these chronic diseases is a challenge for health professionals. In recent years, progress has been made thanks to molecular biology with the development of innovative therapies, for example, new drugs, cellular therapy, etc. [3–5]. They also benefit from major advances in technologies (e.g., sensors, infusion systems, connected objects, etc.) and in artificial intelligence (AI) (e.g., Big Data analysis, deep learning, etc.) [6]. Combined with the information and communication technologies (ICT) and the social and educational sciences, these technological advances and derived tools will probably revolutionize the care of chronic diseases with an optimization of the management [7].

This chapter focuses on actual as well as future technologies and noninvasive devices used in clinical routine at the service of the patients with chronic disease, with the example of diabetes and CHF.

2. Noninvasive sensors for glucose equilibration

Several studies have demonstrated that the external rapid analogue infusion pump associated with the Flash Glucose Monitoring™ system (Abbott Laboratories) (**Figure 1**) is currently the reference management for patients undergoing intensive insulin therapy [9]. In particular, these studies have documented the benefits on HbA1c, the frequency of acute hypoglycemic and hyperglycemic episodes,

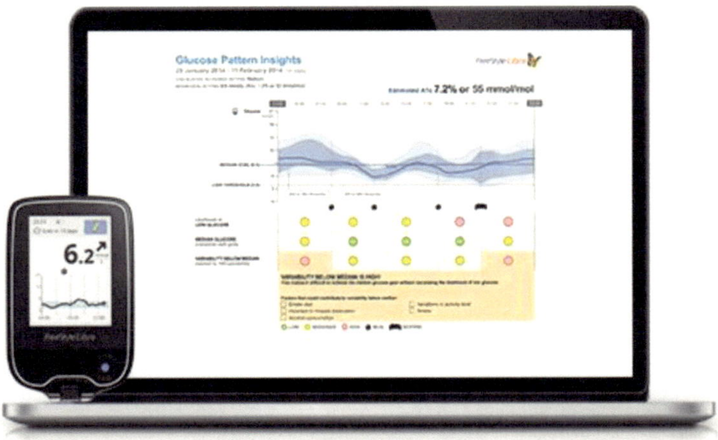

Figure 1.
Flash Glucose Monitoring™ system from Abbott Laboratories (adapted from [8]).

For the diabetic patient, self-monitoring with a capillary blood glucose meter has long been the only way to understand his or her blood glucose control [10]. This self-monitoring gives a more or less truncated reflection of glycemic control (subject to interpretation) and above all allows the patient to adapt his insulin administration. In this setting, Holter glycemia, followed by real-time continuous glucose measurement in the 2000s, revolutionized our vision of glycemic control [6, 10].

In recent years, noninvasive connected sensors measuring interstitial glucose continuously have become more accurate, gradually freeing themselves from calibration constraints (e.g., FreeStyle Libre™, Abbott Laboratories) or from drug interference (e.g., paracetamol), operating for longer and longer (15 days–6 months) and becoming more discreet by placing themselves under the skin (Eversense™, Senseonics/Roche Diabetes Care) [10, 11]. The improvement in their accuracy (meaning mean absolute relative difference [MARD], from 16–20% to 10–14%) allows direct adaptation of insulin without concomitant control of capillary blood glucose levels [11].

3. Noninvasive sensors for glucose self-management

Clinical studies have validated this method, which replaces the classic capillary self-monitoring of blood glucose in the management of patients treated with intensive insulin therapy. Controlled clinical studies have shown the efficacy of these devices on the improvement of HbA1c, associated with a decrease in the time spent in hypoglycemia, in T1D under external pump, but also under multi-injection (Dexcom STS™ System, Dexcom, Inc.) [11]. In addition, their efficacy has also been confirmed in T2D, in pregnant women and in children [12].

The connection of the sensors and the possible sharing of data (Dexcom G5™ Mobile, Dexcom, Inc.) allows a joint analysis of these data by the patient, the parents of a child, the doctor, or the nurse, thus avoiding, thanks to rapid adaptation of the treatment, deterioration in glycemic control. Interstitial glucose data, glycemic variability, and time spent in the target defined for a patient complete the old "hard" criteria of HbA1c and frequency of hypoglycemia.

In some industrialized countries (e.g., in France), the reimbursement by health insurance companies of these devices (e.g., FreeStyle™ Libre, Abbott laboratories) and the soon-to-be-announced reimbursement of sensors coupled to external pumps for highly unstable type 1 diabetic patients opens the way to another modality of the concept of glycemic control assessment [10].

4. Intelligent insulin pumps

For type 1 diabetic and numerous type 2 diabetic patients (e.g., with cardiovascular complications), insulin therapy is the necessary treatment. In this setting, fast or slow insulin analogues are usually administered subcutaneously, with one or more injections per day (e.g., multiple injections in intensive therapy) [4, 9]. In recent years, progress has been made with the development of ultrafast analogues (aspart Fiasp™, Novo Nordisk laboratory, recently launched on the French market), which allow the maximum peak action to be advanced and reduce the duration of action and therefore the quantity of insulin "on board," by about 10 minutes [4]. Nevertheless, the limitations of subcutaneous administration remain related to the still too long insulin kinetics, the reproducibility of imperfect absorption, and the absence of a first hepatic passage that is physiological.

In this context, studies have been carried out with the intraperitoneal route of administration. Compared to the subcutaneous route, this latter improves the HbA1c and is associated with a decrease in the frequency of severe hypoglycemia [13]. The outer surface of the peritoneum appears to be a promising site, and some bioartificial pancreases already use this route (e.g., BAir™, Beta-O2 Technologies and MailPan™ [for Macrocroencapsulation of Pancreatic ILôts], Defymed Company), with kinetic and metabolic results comparable to those of the intraperitoneal route [10]. An access port device allows for optimized insulin delivery either by an external pump or by injections. On this model, the device ExOlin™ (Defymed Company) is under development [14]. ExOlin™ is a medical device for the physiological delivery of insulin. ExOlin™ allows instantaneous intraperitoneal (IP) injection of insulin by simple subcutaneous injection (via an external connection to a syringe, pen, insulin pump, etc.). It includes a biocompatible, non-biodegradable membrane that is permeable to insulin but impermeable to the tissues of the recipient.

The connection of the Enlite™ sensor to the MiniMed Veo™ and 640G™ pumps (Medtronic Company) allows the automatic stopping of insulin infusion when a low interstitial glucose concentration is detected or predicted, dramatically reducing the occurrence of severe hypoglycemia (**Figure 2**) [9].

The recent reimbursement by the health insurance of this system in certain poorly balanced T1D patients, subject to severe hypoglycemia under insulin therapy by pump and adapted self-monitoring, allows for management within the framework of the care of this precursor of the "artificial pancreas."

Several "bolus calculators" have been developed, especially for the insulin pumps, offering a bolus dose by coupling the current blood glucose level and a predetermined insulin/glucose ratio [7]. Nowadays, these systems have been replaced by new intelligent systems based on algorithms (AI) [7, 12].

These latter make it possible to propose a real adaptation of prandial and basal doses by integrating several parameters (glycaemia, insulin sensitivity, etc.) specific to the patient phenotype (personalized medicine). Self-learning, they are specifically adapted to the patient's history of glycemic variations. They have shown their effectiveness on HbA1c, without increasing hypoglycemia, especially when coupled with nursing "coaching" (Diabeo™, Sanofi Laboratory) [16]. This system is currently approved within the framework of telemedicine [7]. Coupled with an external 670G™ pump (Medtronic Company), other algorithms already allow automatic adaptation of basal rates, with the patient managing only bolus doses [12].

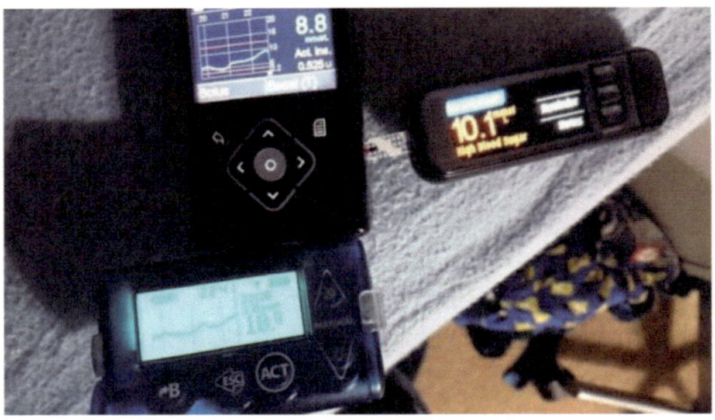

Figure 2.
Enlite™ sensor and MiniMed Veo™ 640G™ pumps from Medtronic Company (adapted from [15]).

5. Artificial pancreas for glycemic management

The artificial pancreas device system is a system of devices that closely mimics the glucose regulating function of a healthy pancreas [17]. Most artificial pancreas consists of three types of devices: a continuous glucose monitoring system (CGM); an insulin infusion pump; and a blood glucose device. A computer-controlled algorithm connects the CGM and insulin infusion pump to allow continuous communication between the two devices. An artificial pancreas device system not only monitors glucose levels in the body but also automatically adjusts the delivery of insulin to reduce high blood glucose levels (hyperglycemia) and minimize the incidence of low blood glucose (hypoglycemia) with little or no input from the patient "the diabetic patient's dream." Its efficacy had been proven in 2015 in one prospective study (ambulatory care of diabetic patients) and confirmed in a recent meta-analysis (24 studies including 585 patients) [17, 18]. This later had documented a significant improvement in the time spent in the target, the reduction of HbA1c and mean blood glucose, without an increase in hypoglycemia [18].

To date, the artificial pancreas is based on a closed-loop insulin delivery system, integrating AI. Most of these devices are mono-hormonal (insulin) and semiautomatic, with the patient manually reporting food intake and physical activity. Many of these devices are expected to be quickly brought to market (e.g., Diabeloop™ from Medtech Company) [19].

The limitations of single-hormonal subcutaneous devices are related to sensor latency, kinetics of interstitial glucose changes, and reproducibility of peripheral administration of subcutaneous insulin. In this setting, the bi-hormonal approach (insulin-glucagon) poses technical problems, as the stability of glucagon and the necessity of double reserves, but seems interesting to avoid hypoglycemia, especially during physical exercise [17, 18].

The addition of amylin or glucagon-like peptide-1 (GLP1) receptor analogue improves post-meal blood glucose levels by decreasing glucagon secretion; future years should make it possible to clarify the place of these molecules in the artificial pancreas.

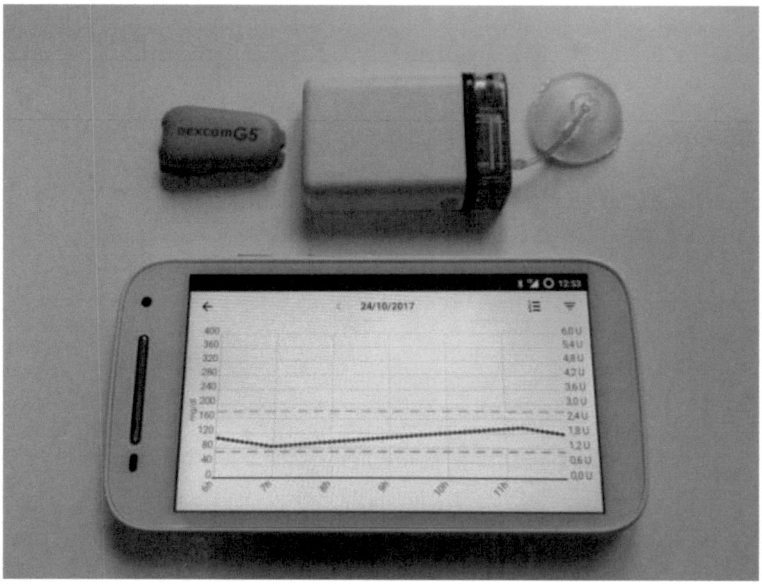

Figure 3.
Diabeloop™ from Medtech Company (adapted from [22]).

Another approach would be to operate other sites that combine sensors and insulin delivery. A study combining a subcutaneous sensor and intraperitoneal insulin infusion showed better regulation of post-meal periods [20]. Intraperitoneal insulin, which is more physiological, could improve problems related to meals and physical activity. Projects to miniaturize the implantable system and reduce its cost are all assets for make it an attractive alternative.

Improving the skills and the capacities of algorithms, by using the database setup (Big Data analysis), optimizing their self-learning capacity and their patient-specific adaptation capacity, and supplementing their information with multiple sensors collecting parameters other than blood glucose levels could allow early detection of food intake, physical activity, stress, and adaptation of the system to specific situations (children, pregnancies, highly unstable diabetes) [21]. The connection of the system to a telemedicine and coaching platform is an evolution that is already underway in the system Diabeloop™ (**Figure 3**).

6. Telemonitoring in the setting of diabetes and chronic heart failure

Over the last 10 years, new-generation telemedicine projects and studies have been developed in the setting of chronic disease management, particularly in the case of telemonitoring [7, 23]. Compared to the first projects, most of these projects incorporate self-administered medical questionnaires or forms on symptoms and signs of diabetes or chronic heart failure (CHF) decompensation; tools for medical education, particularly disease self-appropriation, food hygiene, and physical activity; tools for patient motivation; tools for therapeutic and hygiene observance; tool to remote comorbidities (e.g., arterial hypertension, obesity, dyslipidemia); tools for interaction between the patient and healthcare professionals like telephone support centers, tablets, and Web sites (e.g., Edu@com project for diabetes and e-care project for CHF) (respectively, **Figures 4** and 5) [7, 23].

6.1 Telemonitoring in the setting of diabetes

In the setting of diabetes, the analysis of first-generation projects and studies shows that remote monitoring showed improvements in control of blood glucose

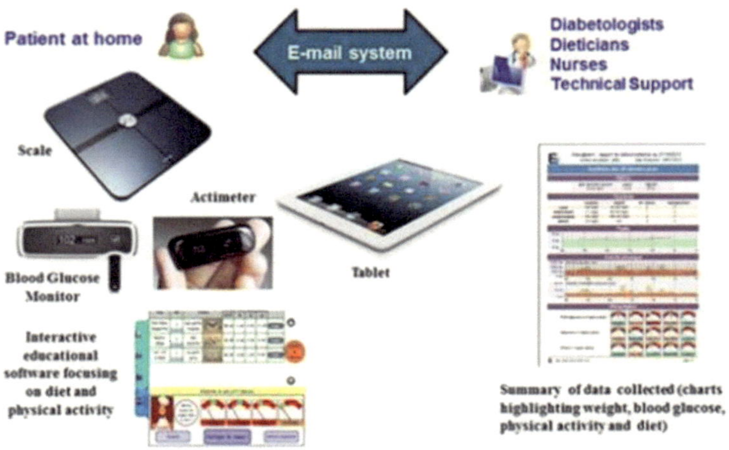

Figure 4.
Telemedicine project for diabetic patients: Educ@dom (adapted from [24]).

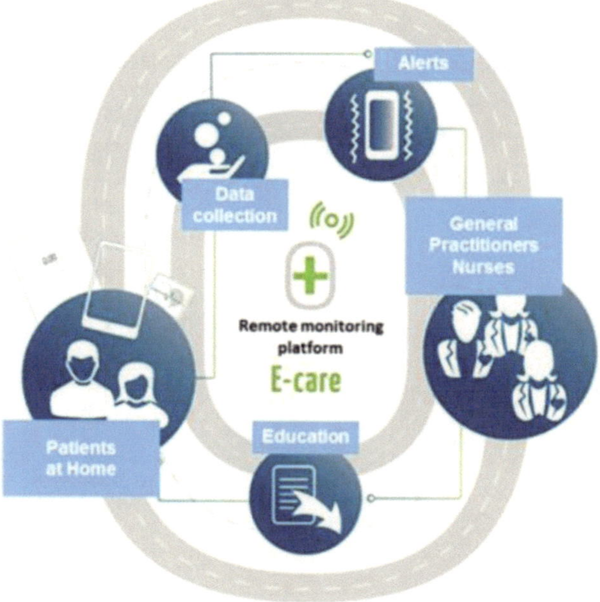

Figure 5.
Telemedicine project for patients with chronic heart failure: e-care (adapted from [12]).

level, significant reduction in HbA1c; better appropriation of the disease by patients; greater adherence to therapeutic and hygiene-dietary measures; positive impact on comorbidities (arterial hypertension, weight, dyslipidemia); better patient's quality of life; and at least, good receptiveness by patients and patient empowerment [7, 23]. Moreover, a cost-effectiveness analysis found a potential of medical economy.

However to date, the magnitude of its effects remains debatable, especially with the variation in patients' characteristics (e.g., background, ability for self-management, and medical condition), sample selection, and approach for treatment of control groups.

Over the last years, new-generation telemedicine projects and studies have emerged in the setting of T1D and T2D [23, 25–27]. They support transmission and remote interpretation of patients' data for follow-up and preventive interventions. **Table 1** lists the characteristics of the telemonitoring studies conducted in the field of diabetes during the period from 2010 to 2015 (**Table 1**) [23, 25–27]. These new-generation telemedicine projects are often known as "telemedicine 2.0" projects, given that they all utilize new ICT and the Web (tools for the "e-Health 2.0") [27].

These projects rely on the standard connected tools for monitoring diabetes, such as glucose meters, BP, heart rate monitors, weighing scales, and pulse oximeters, which relay the collected information via Bluetooth, 3G, or 4G [7, 28]. They include continuous glycemic monitoring solution and often a video call.

The development of practical chemical sensors to monitor parameters, although less mature, is also feasible. However, some external glucose pumps for the chronic management of diabetes also contain chronic intermediate-term (i.e., several days) subcutaneous glucose monitoring capability. The ability of such chemical sensors to augment other device monitoring capabilities for heart failure or other risks will require investigation.

Name of the study	Results
The Utah remote monitoring project ($n = 109$)	Principal criteria: • Mean HbA1c had decreased from 9.73% at baseline to 7.81% at the end of the program ($p < 0.0001$) • Systolic blood pressure (BP) had decreased from 130.7 mmHg at baseline to 122.9 mmHg at the end ($p = 0.0001$) Secondary criteria: • Low-density lipoprotein content had decreased from 103.9 mg/dL at baseline to 93.7 mg/dL at the end ($p = 0.0263$) • Knowledge of diabetes and arterial hypertension have increased significantly ($p < 0.001$ for both) • Patient engagement and medication adherence also have improved, but not significantly • Per questionnaires at study end, patients felt the telemonitoring program had been useful
Randomized trial on home telemonitoring for the management of metabolic and cardiovascular risk in patients with type 2 diabetes ($n = 302$)	Principal criteria: • Mean HbA1c difference of 0.33 ± 0.1 ($p = 0.001$) has been observed between the telemonitoring compared and the control group. The proportion of patients reaching the target of HbA1c (HbA1c <7.0%) had been higher in the telemonitoring group than in the control group after 6 months, 33.0 vs. 18.7% ($p = 0.009$), and 12 months, 28.1 vs. 18.5% ($p = 0.07$) • No difference had been registered for body weight, BP, and lipid profile Secondary criteria: • For quality of life (evaluated with the 36-item short-form health survey), significant differences in favor of the telemonitoring group, as for physical functioning ($p = 0.01$) and mental health ($p = 0.005$) • On an economic level, a lower number of specialist visits was reported in the telemedicine group: incidence rate ratio of 0.72 (95% confidence interval: 0.51–1.01; $p = 0.06$)
Study assessed the utility and cost-effectiveness of an automated diabetes remote monitoring and management system (DMRS) ($n = 98$)	Principal criteria: • No significant difference for mean HbA1c between the DRMS and control groups at 3 months, 7.60 vs. 8.10%, and at 6 months, 8.10 vs. 7.90% (p = ns) Secondary criteria: • Changes from baseline to 6 months have been not statistically significant for self-reported medication adherence • Changes of diabetes-specific quality of life have been not significantly registered, except for the daily quality of life-social/vocational concern subscale score ($p = 0.04$)

Name of the study	Results
Telescot diabetes pragmatic multicenter randomized controlled trial (n = 321)	Principal criteria: • The mean (SD) HbA1c at follow-up was 7.92% in the intervention group vs. 8.36% in the usual care group. For primary analysis, adjusted mean HbA1c was 0.51% lower (95% CI: 0.22–0.81% (principal criterion) (p = 0·0007)) Secondary criteria: • Adjusted mean ambulatory systolic BP has been 3.06 mmHg lower (95% CI: 0.56–5.56 mmHg, p = 0.017), and mean ambulatory diastolic BP has been 2.17 mmHg lower (95% CI: 0.62–3.72, p = 0.006) among people in the intervention group when compared with usual care after adjustment • No significant differences were identified between groups in terms of weight, treatment pattern, and adherence to medication or quality of life • The number of telephone calls was greater between nurses and patients in the intervention compared with control group, rate ratio of 7.50 (95% CI: 4.45–12.65, p < 0.0001), but no other significant differences between groups in use of health services were identified between groups

Table 1.
Results of the telemonitoring studies conducted in the field of diabetes during the period from 2010 to 2015 [23, 25–27].

6.2 Telemonitoring in the setting of chronic heart failure

Over the last 10 years, several new-generation telemedicine projects and trials have emerged in the era of CHF, particularly in Europe [29]. These projects have main objectives: the prevention and treatment of HF exacerbations and the promotion of self-empowerment. Main projects are listed in **Table 2**.

Most of these projects rely on the usual connected tools for monitoring HF, such as blood pressure meters, heart rate monitor, weighing scales, and pulse oximeters, which relay the information collected via Bluetooth, 3G, or 4G [7, 29]. They also incorporate self-administered medical questionnaires or forms (symptoms and signs of HF); tools for medical education, particularly disease self-appropriation, food hygiene, and physical activity; tools for patient motivation; tools for therapeutic and hygiene observance; and tools for interaction between the patient and healthcare professionals like telephone support centers, tablets, and Web sites [29].

Telemonitoring can also be divided in passive or automated, typical of implantable invasive devices that send either sporadically or continuously data to the receiving physician, and active, where, on the contrary, noninvasive devices involve an action or a self-measurement (e.g., blood pressure measurement) that a patient needs to accomplish. While the role of implantable telemonitoring devices for multiparameters or cardiac hemodynamic activity monitoring has been recently established as an effective way to prevent frequent hospitalizations, the role of noninvasive methods for the remote monitoring of CHF patients is still under debate. In this review, we will concentrate, in specific, on the role of external devices and of the electrocardiography for the remote monitoring of CHF patients.

Name of the study	Results
The Trans-European Network—home-care management system (n = 426)	Compared to standard care alone, mortality and rehospitalization rates were shown lower in the groups receiving either telemonitoring or nurse telephone support, without any statistically significant differences between both intervention groups
The BEAT-HF study (n = 437)	All-cause readmissions within 180 days post-discharge occurred in 50.8% (363 of 715) patients from the intervention group versus 49.2% (355 of 722) of those from the control group (adjusted hazard ratio, 1.03 [95% CI: 0.88–1.20]; p = 0.74)
The TIM-HF (n = 710)	All-cause mortality rate (primary end point) was 8.4 per 100 patient-years of follow-up in the telemedicine group and 8.7 per 100 patient-years of follow-up in the standard care group, without significant difference (OR: 0.97 [95% CI: 0.67–1.41]; p = 0.87)
The Telemedical Interventional Management in Heart Failure II (TIM-HF2) (n = 1570)	The percentage of days lost due to unplanned cardiovascular hospital admissions and all-cause death was 4.88% (95% CI: 4.55–5.23) in the remote patient management group versus 6.64% (6.19–7.13) in the standard care group (ratio 0.80, 95% CI: 0.65–1; p = 0.0460)

Table 2.
Results of the telemonitoring studies conducted in the field of chronic heart failure during the period from 2005 to 2018 [7, 29].

In the context of CHF, the number and variety of physiologic sensors and the useful clinical parameters derived from those sensors is likely to continue to increase rapidly [29]. For example, in addition to the capabilities described above, future devices may include additional sensors to track respiration parameters (including rate, minute ventilation, and perhaps apnea and dyspnea detection), tissue perfusion (via optical sensors), cardiac output and stroke volume (via impedance acute ischemia or myocardial infarction via S-T segment monitoring), electrical alternant, and heart rate turbulence. Indeed some recently released devices already contain some of these fascinating capabilities. To date, several projects include BNP monitoring, ECG monitoring, and even a video call [6, 29, 30].

Recently, the TIM-HF2 study is the first to well document the interest of telemedicine in the CHF field, resulting in clinically relevant outcomes with statistical significance (**Table 2**) [31]. In fact, the percentage of days lost due to unplanned cardiovascular hospital admissions and all-cause death was 4.88% (95% CI: 4.55–5.23) in the remote patient management group versus 6.64% (6.19–7.13) in the standard care group (ratio 0.80, 95% CI: 0.65–1; p = 0.0460). Patients assigned to remote patient management lost a mean of 17.8 days (95% CI: 16.6–19.1) per year compared with 24.2 days (95% CI: 22.6–26) per year for patients assigned to standard care. The all-cause death rate was 7.86 (95% CI: 6.14–10.10) per 100 person-years of follow-up in the remote patient management group versus 11.34 (95% CI: 9.21–13.95) per 100 person-years of follow-up in the standard care group (hazard ratio [HR] 0.70, 95% CI: 0.5–0.96; p = 0.0280) (**Figure 6**) [31].

Cardiovascular mortality did not significantly differ between both groups (HR 0.671, 95% CI: 0.45–1.01; p = 0.056).

For this TIM-HF2 care strategy, the key component was a well-structured telemedical center with physicians and HF nurses ("coordination center") available 24 hours a day and every day a week, able to act promptly according to the individual patient risk profile [7, 31]. The actions taken by the telemedical center staff included changes in medication and admission to hospital, as needed, in addition to educational activities.

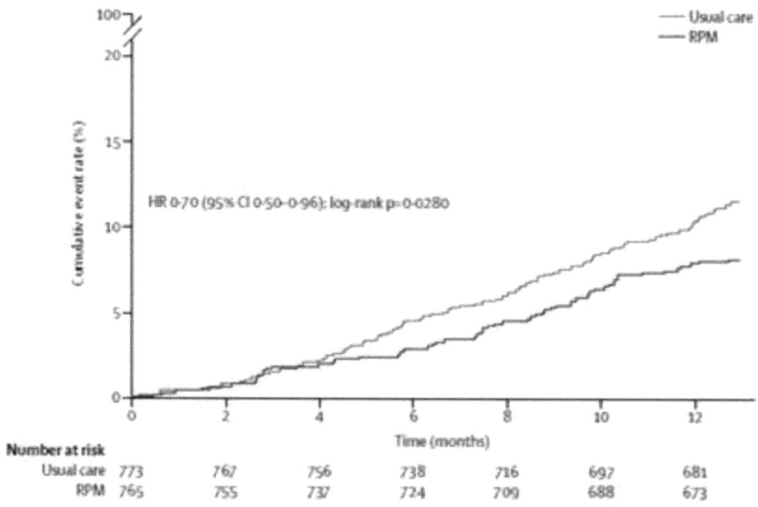

Figure 6.
TIM-HF2 trial (n = 1515). Rate of cumulative events in patients randomly assigned to remote patient management (n = 796) or usual care (n = 775) (adapted from [31]).

7. Artificial intelligence for diabetes and chronic heart failure management

In recent years, several informatic solutions or tools have been developed and used to optimize the management of chronic diseases as diabetes or CHF, for example, artificial neural network (ANN) algorithms, data mining software, and ontology [6, 7]. In this context, three clinical datasets are of particular interest: patients' phenotype; patients' electronic medical records containing physicians' notes, laboratory test results, and other information on diseases, treatments, and epidemiology that may be of interest for association studies and predictive modeling on prognosis and drug responses; and literature knowledge including rules and/or diabetes or CHF management [7, 32].

7.1 Artificial intelligence in telemonitoring in the setting of diabetes

In the setting of diabetes, two telemedicine projects use AI in order to be able, firstly, to adjust the blood glucose level to the patient's activity (software Diabeo™, Sanofi Laboratory) [16] and, secondly, to predict patient risks of diabetes decompensation [33]. In this later situation, the cloud-based software aggregates, cleans, and analyzes patient data to allow for identifying patterns that may indicate potential risks and provide predictive insights on healthcare outcomes, as the software MyPredi™ (Predimed Technology Company) [7, 33].

In the TeleSage study, T1D patients were randomized to usual quarterly follow-up (G1), home use of a smartphone recommending insulin doses (Diabeo™ software) with quarterly visits (G2), or use of the smartphone with short teleconsultations every 2 weeks but no visit until point end (G3) [12, 21]. At 6-month, the mean HbA1c level is 8.41 ± 1.04% in G3 versus 8.63 ± 1.07% in G2 versus 9.10 ± 1.16% in G1 (p = 0.0019 for G1–G3 comparison) (**Figure 7**) [16, 26]. The Diabeo™ system gave a 0.91% (0.60–1.21) improvement in HbA1c over controls and a 0.67% (0.35–0.99) reduction when used without teleconsultation. There was no difference in the frequency of hypoglycemic episodes or in medical time spent for hospital or telephone consultations. However, patients in G1 and G2 spent nearly 5 hours more than G3 patients attending hospital visits.

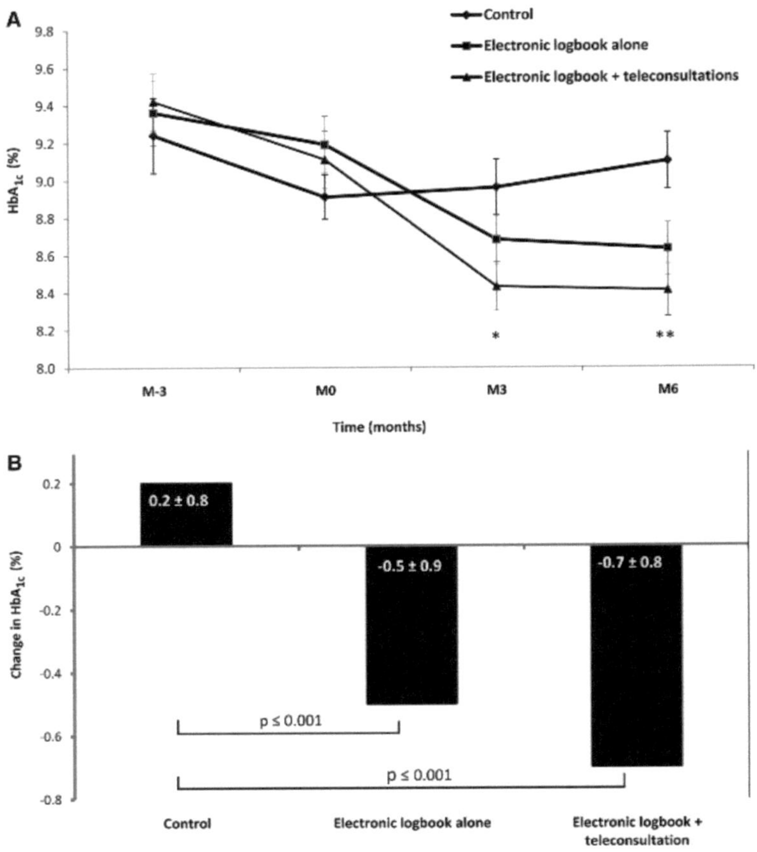

Figure 7.
Efficacy of the software Diabeo™, licensed by Sanofi Laboratory (adapted from [21]). (A) HbA1c values (means ± SE), from 3 months before baseline to month 6. $^{*}p = 0.0103$, $^{**}p = 0.0019$ *compared with control group. (B) Change in HbA1c values (means ± SE) from baseline to month 6.*

The DIABETe telemonitoring project has been developed and designed to optimize home monitoring of diabetic patients by detecting, via a telemonitoring 2.0 platform, situations with a risk of decompensation of diabetes and its complications (e.g., myocardial infarction or CHF), the latter ultimately leading to hospitalization [33]. The AI of the DIABETe platform (MyPredi™) automatically generates indicators of chronic disease deterioration, that is, "warning alerts" for any chronic disease worsening, particularly diabetes, its macrovascular complications, and cardiovascular comorbidities (e.g., arterial hypertension and CHF). For the patient, these situations may lead to hospitalization if not treated appropriately. To our knowledge, this is one of the first projects that use AI in addition to ICT. The platform comprises connected nonintrusive medical sensors, a touchscreen tablet connected by Wi-Fi, and a router or 3G/4G, rendering it possible to interact with the patient and provide education on treatment, diet, and lifestyle (**Figure 8**) [7, 33].

The telemonitoring platform used in DIABETe was first validated in a monocentric study conducted in the Strasbourg University Hospital, carried out as part of the e-care project, primarily focused on the problem of CHF [34].

7.2 Artificial intelligence in telemonitoring in the setting of chronic heart failure

e-Care has been initially developed and designed to optimize home monitoring of CHF patients by detecting, via a telemonitoring 2.0 platform, situations with a risk of cardiac decompensation and rehospitalization. Between February 2014

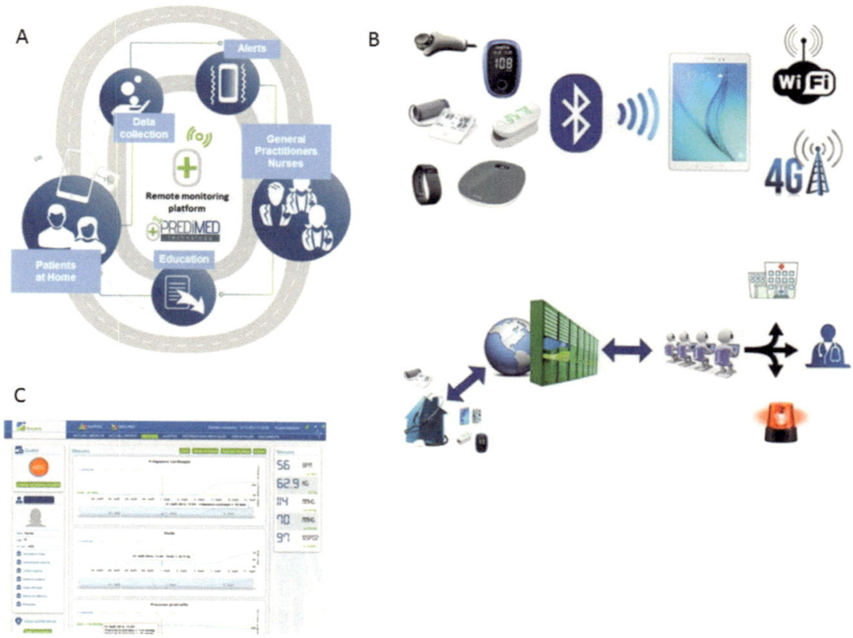

Figure 8.
Intelligent telemonitoring project on diabetes and/or chronic heart failure management. (A) The system is based on an inference engine and a medical ontology for personalized synchronous or asynchronous analysis of data specific to each patient and, if necessary, the sending of an artificial intelligence-generated alert (MyPredi™). (B) The platform comprises connected nonintrusive medical sensors, a touchscreen tablet connected by Wi-Fi, and a router or 3G/4G, rendering it possible to interact with the patient and provide education on treatment, diet, and lifestyle. (C) The system involves a server that hosts the patient's data and a secure Internet portal to which the patient and hospital- and non-hospital-based healthcare professionals can connect.

and April 2015, 175 patients were included into the e-care project [35]. During this period, the e-care platform was used on a daily basis by patients and healthcare professionals, according to a defined protocol of use specific to each patient. The mean age of these patients was 72 years, and the ratio of men to women is 0.7. The patients suffered from multiple concomitant diseases, with a mean Charlson index of 4.1. The five main diseases were CHF in more than 60% of subjects, anemia in more than 40%, atrial fibrillation in 30%, T2D in 30%, and chronic obstructive pulmonary disease in 30%. During the study, 1500 measurements were taken in these 175 patients, which resulted in the e-care system generating 700 alerts in 68 patients [35]. Some 107 subjects (61.1%) had no alerts upon follow-up. Follow-up data analysis of these 107 patients revealed that they exhibited no clinically significant events that might eventually have led to hospitalization. Analysis of the warning alerts showed that the e-care platform automatically and nonintrusively detected any worsening of the patient's health, particularly HF decompensation (between 2 and 9 days), with a sensitivity, specificity, and positive and negative predictive values of 100, 72, 90, and 100%, respectively. Both the healthcare professionals and patients, even the frailest, used the e-care system without difficulty until the end of the study. For nonautonomous patients, the system was employed by a nurse in addition to her other assigned tasks, such as washing and administering medication, or by close ones and family members [35].

To date, an enhanced version of the e-care platform and the AI (MyPredi™) will be experimented in the homes of CHF patients as part of a project called PRADO INCADO [7]. PRADO is a French program to support patients returning home after hospital, while PRADO INCADO will specifically target HF patients in this setting. Over a period of several months, it will follow 300 patients with NYHA Stages I–IV

HF using the PRADO organizational model for CHF patients developed by the national health insurance.

8. Conclusions

This review supports the efficacy of numerous current and new technologies and noninvasive tools for a better management of patients with chronic diseases, particularly diabetic patients and patients with CHF. Nevertheless, in chronic diseases, the magnitude of its effects remains to date debatable or to be consolidated, especially with the variation in patients' characteristics and methods of experimentation and in terms of medical and economic objectives.

To our opinion, innovative technologies based on AI (machine learning, Big Data) are going to build the future of chronic disease, and they invent the medicine of tomorrow.

Competing interest

M. Hajjam is the scientific director of Predimed Technology (www.predimed-technology.fr). All other authors have declared that no competing interests exist.

Funding

Grants from the Agence Régionale de Santé du Grand Est (ARS).

Consent and ethical approval

Not applicable.

Ethical approval

Not applicable.

Guarantor

EA.

Author details

Emmanuel Andrès[1,2]*, Nathalie Jeandidier[3], Samy Talha[2,4], Abrar-Ahmad Zulfiqar[1,2], Laurent Meyer[3], Noel Lorenzo Villalba[1], Thibault Bahougne[3], Mohamed Hajjam[5] and Amir Hajjam El Hassani[6]

1 Service de Médecine Interne, Diabète et Maladies Métaboliques de la Clinique Médicale B, Hôpitaux Universitaires de Strasbourg, Strasbourg Cedex, France

2 Equipe de recherche EA 3072 "Mitochondrie, Stress oxydant et Protection musculaire", Faculté de Médecine de Strasbourg, Université de Strasbourg (Unistra), Strasbourg, France

3 Service d'Endocrinologie et de Diabétologie de la Clinique Médicale B, Hôpitaux Universitaires de Strasbourg, Strasbourg, France

4 Service de Physiologie et d'Explorations Fonctionnelles, Hôpitaux Universitaires de Strasbourg, Strasbourg, France

5 Predimed Technology, Strasbourg, France

6 Equipe de recherche EA 4662 "Nanomédecine, Imagerie, Thérapeutiques", Université de Technologie de Belfort-Montbéliard (UTBM), Belfort-Montbéliard, France

*Address all correspondence to: emmanuel.andres@chru-strasbourg.fr

IntechOpen

© 2020 The Author(s). Licensee IntechOpen. This chapter is distributed under the terms of the Creative Commons Attribution License (http://creativecommons.org/licenses/by/3.0), which permits unrestricted use, distribution, and reproduction in any medium, provided the original work is properly cited.

References

[1] Available from: http://invs.santepubliquefrance.fr/publications/etat_sante_2017/ESP2017_Ouvrage_complet_vdef.pdf [Accessed: April 2019]

[2] Available from: http://www.has-sante.fr/portail/upload/docs/application/pdf/2012-04/guideparcoursdesoinsicweb.pdf [Accessed: April 2019]

[3] Jessup M, Brozena S. Heart failure. The New England Journal of Medicine. 2003;**348**:2007-2018

[4] Nathan DM. Diabetes: Advances in diagnosis and treatment. Journal of the American Medical Association. 2015;**314**:1052-1062

[5] Bartlett ST, Markmann JF, Johnson P, et al. Report from IPITA-TTS opinion leaders meeting on the future of B-cell replacement. Transplantation. 2016;**100**(Suppl. 2):S1-S44

[6] Rjeily CB, Badr G, El Hassani AH, Andrès E. Medical data mining for heart diseases and the future of sequential mining. Machine Learning Paradigms: Advances in Data Analytics. 2018;**149**:71-99

[7] Andrès E, Hajjam M, Talha S, et al. Télémédecine dans le domaine de l'insuffisance cardiaque. État des lieux et focus Sur le projet de télémédecine 2.0 E-care. Perspectives dans le domaine de la diabétologie. Médecine des maladies Métaboliques. 2018;**12**:224-231

[8] https://www.google.com/search?q=Flash+Glucose+Monitoring+system+(Abbott+Laboratory)&client=firefox-b-ab&source=lnms&tbm=isch&sa=X&ved=0ahUKEwimtoSBsMLfAhUEIVAKHUhUD1cQ_AUIECgD&biw=1920&bih=954

[9] Benhamou PY, Lablanche S. Diabète de type 1: Perspectives technologiques. Maharashtra Centre for Entrepreneurship Development. 2018;**92**:11-16

[10] Rodbard D. Continuous glucose monitoring: A review of recent studies demonstrating improved glycemic outcomes. Diabetes Technology & Therapeutics. 2017;**19**(Suppl. 3):S25-S37

[11] Borot S, Benhamou PY, Atlan C, et al. Practical implementation, education and interpretation guidelines for continuous glucose monitoring: A French position statement. Diabetes & Metabolism. 2018;**44**:61-72

[12] Biester T, Kordonouri O, Holder M, et al. "Let the algorithm do the work": Reduction of hypo-glycemia using sensor–augmented pump therapy with predictive insulin suspension (SmartGuard) in pediatric type 1 diabetes patients. Diabetes Technology & Therapeutics. 2017;**19**:173-182

[13] Barrientos R, Baltrusch S, Sigrist S, Legeay G, Belcourt A, Lenzen S. Kinetics of insulin secretion from MIN6 pseudoislets after encapsulation in a prototype device of a bioartificial pancreas. Hormone and Metabolic Research. 2009;**41**:5-9

[14] Available from: https://www.defymed.com/mailpan/ [Accessed: 27 April 2018]

[15] https://www.google.com/search?client=firefox-b-ab&biw=1920&bih=954&tbm=isch&sa=1&ei=SQgmXLq4JsnkkgWAq53wCw&q=MiniMed+Veo+and+640G+&oq=MiniMed+Veo+and+640G+&gs_l=img.3.50784.53946.54601.0.0.0.0.72.188.3.0.1.gws-wiz-img.UjQ_2YH35qw#imgrc=h50L-In2D0oL2M

[16] Jeandidier N, Chaillous L, Franc S, et al. DIABEO app software and telemedicine versus usual follow-up in the treatment of diabetic patients:

Protocol for the TELESAGE randomized controlled trial. JMIR Research Protocols. 2018;7:e66

[17] Castle JR, DeVries JH, Kovatchev B. Future of automated insulin delivery systems. Diabetes Technology & Therapeutics. 2017;**19**:S67-S72

[18] Bertachi A, Ramkissoon CM, Bondia J, Vehí J. Automated blood glucose control in type 1 diabetes: A review of progress and challenges. Endocrinology, Diabetes and Nutrition. 2018;**65**:172-181

[19] Christiansen SC, Fougner AL, Stavdahl Ø, et al. A review of the current challenges associated with the development of an artificial pancreas by a double subcutaneous approach. Diabetes Therapy. 2017;**8**:489-506

[20] Renard E, Place J, Cantwell M, et al. Closed-loop insulin delivery using a subcutaneous glucose sensor and intraperitoneal insulin delivery: Feasibility study testing a new model for the artificial pancreas. Diabetes Care. 2010;**33**:121-127

[21] Aleppo G, Webb K. Continuous glucose monitoring integration in clinical practice: A stepped guide to data review and interpretation. Journal of Diabetes Science and Technology. 2018;**17**:1-7. DOI: 10.1177/1932296818813581

[22] https://www.google.com/search?q=Diabeloop&client=firefox-b-d&source=lnms&tbm=isch&sa=X&ved=0ahUKEwi__r2qxv_hAhXC5eAKHYg9CoYQ_AUIDygC&biw=1920&bih=954#imgrc=eMwbvNkL9Y9O9M

[23] Andrès E, Talha S, Jeandidier N, Meyer L, Hajjam M, Hajjam A. Telemedicine in chronic diseases: The time of maturity with telemedicine 2.0 in the setting of chronic heart failure and diabetes mellitus! Current Research in Clinical Diabetes and Obesity. 2018;**6**:1-4

[24] https://www.google.com/search?q=telemonitoring+diabetic+patient&client=firefox-b&source=lnms&tbm=isch&sa=X&ved=0ahUKEwj6h92uuMLfAhWPzKQKHclfAhkQ_AUIDigB&biw=1920&bih=918#imgrc=0Eh6raxPEr0VFM

[25] Lindberg I, Torbjørnsen A, Söderberg S, Ribu L. Telemonitoring and health counseling for self-management support of patients with type 2 diabetes: A randomized controlled trial. JMIR Diabetes. 2017;**2**:e10

[26] Charpentier G, Benhamou PY, Dardari D, et al. The Diabeo software enabling individualized insulin dose adjustments combined with telemedicine support improves HbA1c in poorly controlled type 1 diabetic patients: A 6-month, randomized, open-label, parallel-group, multicenter trial (TeleDiab 1 study). Diabetes Care. 2011;**34**:533-539

[27] Van De Belt TH, Engelen L, Berben S, Schoonhoven L. Definition of Health 2.0 and Medicine 2.0: A systematic review. Journal of Medical Internet Research. 2010;**12**:e18

[28] Puricel SG, Ruiz J. Le diabète et l'ère de la télémédecine. Revue Médicale Suisse. 2014;**10**:1246-1248

[29] Andrès E, Talha S, Zulfiqar AA, Hajjam M, Ervé S, Hajjam J, et al. Current researches and new perspectives of telemedicine in chronic heart failure. Journal of Clinical Medicine. 2018;**7**:544. DOI: 10.3390/jcm7120544

[30] Ahmed Benyahia A, Hajjam A, Talha S, Hajjam M, Andrès E, Hilaire V. E-care: évolution ontologique et amélioration des connaissances pour le suivi des insuffisants cardiaques. Medecine Thérapeutique. 2014;**20**:79-86

[31] Koehler F, Koehler K, Deckwart O, Prescher S, Wegscheider K, Kirwan BA,

et al. Efficacy of telemedical interventional management in patients with heart failure (TIM-HF2): A randomised, controlled, parallel-group, unmasked trial. Lancet. 2018;**392**:1047-1057

[32] Mortazavi BJ, Downing NS, Bucholz EM, Dharmarajan K, Manhapra A, Li SX, et al. Analysis of machine learning techniques for heart failure readmissions. Circulation. Cardiovascular Quality and Outcomes. 2016;**9**:629-640

[33] Available from: https://www.predimed-technology.fr/solutions/plateforme-intelligente-my-predi/ [Accessed: 27 April 2019]

[34] Andrès E, Talha S, Hajjam M, Hajjam J, Ervé S, Hajjam A. E-care project: A promising e-plateform for the optimizing management of chronic heart failure and other chronic diseases. Journal of Heart Research. 2015;**1**:39-45

[35] Andrès E, Talha S, Hajjam M, Hajjam J, Ervé S, Hajjam A. Experimentation of 2.0 telemedicine in elderly patients with chronic heart failure: A study prospective in 175 patients. European Journal of Internal Medicine. 2018;**51**:e11-e12

Chapter 3

Primary Health-Care Service Delivery and Accessibility in the Digital Age

Thierry Edoh

Abstract

The primary care is within a health-care system, the first contact and main point for people requiring health and medical care. Patients requiring specialized health and medical care are directed to the appropriate specialists by a general physician (GP) who coordinates the needed specialist care. GPs base their decisions partially on patient-centered information and partially on the results of medical examinations. Many health-IT systems for primary health care are available today. Their first aims are to assist GPs in their daily duties and the patient in collecting his medical data and to self-manage his conditions. IT systems enabling the patient to collect accurate information on his condition to self-manage his condition provide accurate patient-centric data, which shows the potential to outperform patient-centered information, which in turn is based on the patient's personal feeling and perception. Patient-centered information are biased. Beyond providing patient-centric information, health-IT systems can facilitate access to health-care services, increase the quality, efficiency, and effectiveness of health-care services, and can contribute to reducing medical expenses. This chapter aims to paint down the global trend of health-IT systems and the supporting technology. The chapter will further present some existing health-IT systems and discuss their role in the health-care accessibility, particularly in rural regions.

Keywords: health-IT, care accessibility, primary care, patient-centered data, patient-centric data

1. Introduction

Various health information technology (HIT) initiatives emerge today and are part of the strategy defined by each nation to assist health-care professionals in their daily duties as well as to decrease the medical expenses, which keep increasing day by day. High-income countries (HIC) as well as low- and middle-income countries (LMIC) are putting efforts to provide their health-care systems with HIT. Beyond these efforts, researchers are working on innovative HIT to assist the patient in managing his health conditions [1, 2], access to health-care services [3], and to assist general physicians (GP) in their daily duties.

LMIC and rural regions in HIC are mostly medically underserved and thus facing poor access to care services. LMIC rural regions are severely facing poor care access issues. Patients are living very far from care units [4]. Rural regions in HIC

IntechOpen

are mostly suffering from a low rate of physicians providing medical services in these regions [5].

Overall, the primary health-care sector is increasingly being provided with modern information systems that assist medical doctors in their daily duties supporting them in decision-making, diagnosing, prescribing, and remote delivering care service to patients.

eHealth, mHealth, telehealth, and telemedicine are modern HIT-enabled tools aiming to provide better, efficient, and effective care services to the patient. Telehealth and telemedicine enable care service delivery regardless of the time zone, the geographic residence place of the patient, and his medical doctor(s). Rural regions (medically underserved) are mostly taking benefit of these tools supporting remote care [6].

HIT systems collect and provide medical information to medical doctors (MD), to the patient for self-management of his health conditions (for example, glucometer and tensiometer). HIT also processes collected data to assist in decision-making. These data are stored in the so-called "electronic health records—EHR—or electronic medical records—EMR." Evidence has shown the benefits of EMR/EHR. They could reduce prescription errors [7] and enable inter- and extra-organizational information sharing [8]. Beyond decreasing the rate of prescription errors, EMR could support accurate diagnosis making and thus impact the patient's health outcomes.

The objectives of this chapter are to paint the tableau of existing HIT and systems in primary care, which improve access to health-care services, assist health-care professionals in decision-making by providing them with appropriate data at the right time, empower patients toward their conditions (diseases awareness and health literacy), medical document management, etc. This chapter further aims to discuss the state of the art and the future of the HIT.

The remainder of the chapter defines some HIT-related terms (Section Backgrounds and definitions) presents the state of the art in LMIC and HIC. It discusses the future of HIT (Section Discussion and conclusion) and concludes the work in the last section.

2. Backgrounds and definitions

Health information technology (HIT): it is the field of information and communication technology mainly focusing on process automation and medical data processing to support health-care service delivery, patient's self-management, and any other related processes. The main purposes and priorities of implementing HIT are summarized in **Table 1**. Zayas et al. discuss the HIT priorities for the research. Data quality, harmonization, interoperability, storage, integration, and aggregation are the main points that the HIT research has to focus on [9].

eHealth: — stands for electronic health. The term "eHealth" lacks uniformity of definition—*standard definition*—[10]. We define eHealth as the use of information technology and/or systems and electronic devices for health-care service delivery. Furthermore, eHealth mostly focuses on medical informatics and deals with data, while biomedical provides medical devices to support care services. An electronic medical record system is an eHealth system that records patient's medical data. A hospital information system is also an eHealth system that collects, processes, and stores any data related to a hospital as described in **Table 2**.

mHealth: it is a subset of eHealth supported by mobile technology, i.e., mobile network, and mobile devices such as mobile phones and tablets.

The World Health Organization defines mHealth as:

> *mHealth is a component of eHealth. To date, no standardized definition of mHealth has been established. For the purposes of the survey, the Global Observatory for eHealth (GOe) defined mHealth or mobile health as medical and public health practice supported by mobile devices, such as mobile phones, patient monitoring devices, personal digital assistants (PDAs), and other wireless devices. mHealth involves the use and capitalization on a mobile phone's core utility of voice and short messaging service (SMS) as well as more complex functionalities and applications including general packet radio service (GPRS), third and fourth generation mobile telecommunications (3G and 4G systems), global positioning system (GPS), and Bluetooth technology [11].*

Digital health care: while eHealth is dealing with supporting the health and medical care delivery using health-IT, digital health focuses more on the patient and personalized medicine by using digital channels to collect patient's medical data, helping the patient to self-manage his health conditions using digital platforms or tools.

Pos.	Priority	Description
1	Medical data quality	The improvement of the quality of medical data at the point of the collection is very important. Biased or wrong data could negatively impact patient's health outcomes. Today, with the advancement of technology, efforts are put to collect accurate and right data using technology such as RFID, sensors, and camera. The Internet of Things is the widespread paradigm today to autonomously and automatically capture, process, and store medical data.
2	Data harmonization and interoperability	For analytics purposes, data harmonization is needed. However, data harmonization is still challenging. HL7 is a standard that is used to overcome harmonization issues. In health-care systems, many devices using different data formats are being used. In many cases, an intercommunication and data exchange between these devices is mandatory. Therefore, HIT application need to be support any data format (Data interoperability).
3	Data processing and storage	In the digital age, the amount of data produced every day is fast growing. Processing and storing such data are challenging. Big data computing and data sciences provide the framework and technology to face issues related to the fast-growing data.
4	Data sources integration and aggregation	Many data sources are emerged due to the digital age and technology advancement. The advancement of the Internet provides social media data, wearable technology produces many health data, etc. All these data need to be integrated and aggregated.

Table 1.
Priorities of health-IT [9].

Hospital information systems (HIS)	• Electronic medical record systems (EMRs, EHRs, and PHRs)
	• Clinical decision support systems
	• Computerized disease surveillance and monitoring systems
	• Patient's bed management system
	• Health-care professional management system (HR)
	• Drug management systems
	• Health insurance management systems, etc.

Table 2.
Sub-systems of HIS.

3. Existing eHealth and digital health applications categories (state of the art)

This section presents some existing categories of health-IT applications and some concrete developed and deployed health-IT applications. These applications cover the key areas listed above. They are using Internet technology and services and assist in decision-making, etc.

3.1 Categories of health-IT applications

eHealth applications mostly cover the following areas:

1. ***Electronic medical records*** (EMR): it is a sub-set of ***electronic health records*** (EHR) also called federated EMR [12] that includes patient's medical records, digital imaging and archiving systems, e-prescribing, e-booking, and clinical administration systems. Despite that, the use of EMR/EHR could positively impact patient's health outcomes and make the patient care safer [7].

   The adoption of (mobile) patient's medical records is worldwide moderate [11]. Health-care professionals and care units (hospitals, clinics, etc.) possess temporary and non-maintained patient's records. The patient's medical data are dispersed everywhere and thus incomplete at each point. Connected EMR aims at overcoming these issues in bundling the data to a central point.

2. ***Telemedicine and telecare services***: telemedicine is a discipline of health informatics that uses HIT to provide health and medical care service a remote. It covers all fields of common health care such as surgery (telesurgery), cardiology (telecardiology), tele-education, and telediagnostics.

   Telemedicine uses technologies like video streaming, voice IP, etc. Its main purpose is to increase health-care accessibility in regions facing poor access to health care by delivering care services to remote patients. Teleconsultation is the most used telemedicine artifact followed by tele-education and teleassistance. Care specialists can use it to assist less experienced health-care professionals.

3. ***Health information networks*** (HIN): HIN are standards, policies, and services. The objectives of HIN are to secure health information exchange over the Internet. HIN are, therefore, important than medical data, which are sensitive data that need to be protected for reasons such as data integrity prevention.

4. ***Decision support tools***: machine learning/deep learning all sub-sets of artificial intelligence (AI) are being involved in eHealth applications to support decision-making. Decision support tools mostly use patient's data as sources and base the analysis on such data. They ease the data analytics and can assist in event medical prediction.

5. ***Internet-based technologies and services***: the Internet is the data highway that enables data and information exchange as well as communication between the different actors within a health system.

The Internet of Things is an Internet-based technology that enables us to collect data and transfer them over the Internet to a remote server, where the data will be processed.

3.2 Existing applications

The existing applications are shown in **Table 3**.

System designation/country	Description
EpharmacyNet/Benin	EpharmacyNet is developed for African countries to assist patients and health-care professionals in prescribing and purchasing medicine. LMICs are lacking pharmaceutical products. This situation leads to a phenomenon where the patient needs to go to many pharmacies before purchasing the needed medicine.
Mobile HybriCare[1] Mobile electronic data capture (EDC) system/Germany	Allow fast, simple, and cost-effective recording of patient's data in real time.
eReader/Canada + Kenya	A self-measurement blood pressure device to assist the patient with the daily self-management of his blood pressure and cardiologic condition
Health and hospital information systems/Spain	This system provides a platform to manage patient's information
Maternal and child health mobile services/India	This system addresses maternal neonatal and infant mortality issues in India
Teleophthalmology/India	A system that aids primary eye care
Dry blood spot screening/Spain and Brazil	This system supports early diagnosis prevention of diseases

Source: Ref. [13]. [1]*https://www.uni-kassel.de/fb07/?id=38057.*

Table 3.
eHealth systems in primary health care (a digest).

4. Trends and technology supporting eHealth systems

This section will present trends and perspectives in eHealth.

4.1 Supporting technologies

A lot of modern information and communication technologies are emerging and the health-care sector is taking benefit of these technologies. Blockchain (BC), artificial intelligence (AI), and Internet of Things (IoT) are the most emerging technologies that find application in health-care service delivery. Big data computing supports computing the huge amount of medical data which ICT systems are producing day by day.

Through the emerging information technologies like AI and big data analytics, the term "personalized medicine" is becoming more important. We are surrounded by huge medical devices, which pervasively collect gapless medical data. So, collected data are accurate and complete since these devices are becoming precise, sophisticate, and powerful. Nevertheless, eHealth is confronting a critical issue called data interoperability. Purposely, HL7—Health Level 7—, a group of international standards, is provided to overcome any interoperability that could occur during data exchange. HL7-FHIR is the standard on top of HL7 to secure patient's medical data. Blockchain is using today to achieve a similar goal, data protection.

4.2 Medical and health care data records (EMR/EHR)

Despite the moderate implementation and use of electronic medical records to manage patient's medical data, each medical unit has a relatively complete patient's medical data record, which is used to collect and process part of the patient's medical data and. These data are used to deliver adequate care. Unfortunately, these data record systems are not interconnected with other systems beyond the given health center. The patient's data are thus dispersed in many small medical records (partially electronic and partially paper-based). Health records, as the superset of all patient's medical records, do not exist.

4.3 Hospital 4.0 and Health 4.0

The model of Industry 4.0 aims to automatically and autonomously collect patient's medical data within a hospital and process them for efficient and effective medical treatment. It relies on machine-to-machine and human-to-machine interactions.

> *Industry 4.0 aims to emphasize the importance of production technology, supporting information, and the communication technology sector [14].*

Hospital 4.0 is supported by modern technologies like the Internet of Things (machine-to-machine—M2M) technology and paradigm, cloud, and fog computing [15], artificial intelligence (AI), mobile network, etc. It comprehends the AI, precision medicine, and telemedicine [16].

Hospital 4.0 initiatives are emerging in developed countries, while developing countries are still facing a digital divide due to their low technical development level.

Health 4.0 like Hospital 4.0 is inspired by Industry 4.0 [17]. According to Mukherjee (2020),

> *The concept aims for virtualization of services, decentralization of records, and personalization for patients, professionals, and other stakeholders leading to the overall improvement of services, through technology. Driven by networked Electronic Health Record (EHR) systems, Artificial Intelligence (AI), real-time data from wearable devices and body sensor networks, and improved data analytics, Health 4.0 is set to completely metamorphose the health-care industry [17].*

Blockchain technology is also used to support Health 4.0/Hospital 4.0 particularly to secure patient's data and information during a data exchange process. The patient's data can be thus protected again by any manipulation.

4.4 Patient's self-management

Self-management of chronic diseases is a sub-set of Healthcare 4.0. The patient can today self-manage his condition through the data provided by surrounded devices like Google-watch, etc. Many self-management applications and systems exist today.

Patients suffering from chronic diabetes and cardiovascular diseases have various medical devices to track their condition daily. Various electronic data capture (EDC) systems exist today. They assist the patient in tracking and collecting data on their condiction. Those data are used by medical doctors to provide data-driven treatment.

5. Discussion and conclusion

Developing countries are putting effort to implement a huge ehealth system to improve access to health-care services in rural. Their effort to launch ehealth aims to improve the quality of health-care services provided. The role of ehealth in patient's health outcomes and its impacts on the care quality are well documented. However, less-developed countries face structural, infrastructural, and financial as well as manpower issues to implement ehealth systems. Many start-ups are raising today and offer low-cost solutions. In Refs. [11, 13], WHO has shown the trends eHealth/mHealth in low-resource settings. Mobile eHealth is emerging in these parts of the world.

This chapter has summarized the trend in eHealth and has pointed out the technologies that support eHealth today.

Author details

Thierry Edoh
RFW-Universität Bonn, Germany

*Address all correspondence to: oscar.edoh@gmail.com

IntechOpen

© 2020 The Author(s). Licensee IntechOpen. This chapter is distributed under the terms of the Creative Commons Attribution License (http://creativecommons.org/licenses/by/3.0), which permits unrestricted use, distribution, and reproduction in any medium, provided the original work is properly cited.

References

[1] Shire KA, Leimeister JM, editors. Technologiegestützte Dienstleistungsinnovation in der Gesundheitswirtschaft. Wiesbaden: Gabler Verlag; 2012

[2] Yang Z, Kankanhalli A, Ng BY, Lim JTY. Examining the pre-adoption stages of healthcare IT: A case study of vital signs monitoring systems. Information Management. 2015;**52**(4):454-467

[3] Edoh TO, Teege G. Using information technology for an improved pharmaceutical care delivery in developing countries. Study case: Benin. Journal of Medical Systems. 2011;**35**(5):1123-1134

[4] Edoh TO. ICT-Systeme zur Verbesserung der Gesundheitsversorgung in den Gesundheitssystemen der afrikanischen Entwicklungsländern. Fallstudien: Benin. Germany: Universität der Bundeswehr München: Athene-Forschung; 2010

[5] Edoh TO. Advanced Systems for Improved Public Healthcare and Disease Prevention. USA: IGI Global, Medical Information Science Reference (an Imprint of IGI Global); 2018

[6] Edoh TO, Pawar PA, Brügge B, Teege G. A multidisciplinary remote healthcare delivery system to increase health care access, pathology screening, and treatment in developing countries. In: Health Care Delivery and Clinical Science. Concepts, Methodologies, Tools, and Applications, Hershey, PA: IGI Global; 2018. pp. 269-302

[7] Hydari MZ, Telang R, Marella WM. Saving patient Ryan - Can advanced electronic medical records make patient care safer? Management Science. 2019;**65**(5):2041-2059

[8] Adjerid I, Adler-Milstein J, Angst C. Reducing medicare spending through electronic health information exchange: The role of incentives and exchange maturity. Information Systems Research. 2018;**29**(2):341-361

[9] Zayas-Cabán T, Chaney KJ, Rucker DW. National health information technology priorities for research: A policy and development agenda. Journal of the American Medical Informatics Association. 2020;**00**(0):1-6

[10] Engemann C. eHealth. In: Kasprowicz D, Rieger S, editors. Virtualität. Wiesbaden: Springer Fachmedien Wiesbaden; 2020. pp. 361-372

[11] WHO. mHealth: New Horizons for Health through Mobile Technologies. Vol. 3. Geneva: WHO Library Cataloguing-in-Publication Data; 2011

[12] Edoh T. Internet of things in emergency medical care and services. In: Farhadi H, editor. Medical Internet of Things (m-IoT) - Enabling Technologies and Emerging Applications. Vol. 2. London: IntechOpen; 2019. p. 64

[13] World Health Organisation. Compendium of Innovative Health Technologies for Low-Resource Settings: Assistive Devices eHealth Solutions. Geneva: WHO Library Cataloguing-in-Publication Data Compendium; 2013. pp. 1-124

[14] Oztemel E, Gursev S. Literature review of industry 4.0 and related technologies. Journal of Intelligent Manufacturing. 2020;**31**(1):127-182

[15] Aceto G, Persico V, Pescapé A. Industry 4.0 and health: Internet of things, big data, and cloud computing for healthcare 4.0. Journal of Industrial Information Integration. 2020;**18**(100129):1-17

[16] Chen C, Loh EW, Kuo KN, Tam KW. The times they are a-Changin' – Healthcare 4.0 is coming! Journal of Medical Systems. 2020;**44**(2):0-3

[17] Mukherjee P, Singh D. "The opportunities of blockchain in health 4.0," in Blockchain Technology for Industry 4.0, R. da Rosa Righi, A.M. Alberti, and M. Singh, Eds. Singapore: Springer Singapore; 2020, pp. 149-164

Chapter 4

Telemedicine Network in Pediatric Cardiology: The Case of Tuscany Region in Italy

Alessandro Taddei, Pierluigi Festa, Fabrizio Conforti, Giuseppe Santoro, Gianluca Rocchi and Luciano Ciucci

Abstract

Four years ago, a telemedicine project in diagnosis and care of congenital cardiac malformations was developed in Tuscany interconnecting the Heart Hospital of Gabriele Monasterio Tuscany Foundation (FTGM) in Massa with main clinical centers around the region. Both live and store-and-forward tele-echocardiography were implemented, while the FTGM medical record system was applied for collaborative reporting. Mobile medical-grade carts, equipped with videoconferencing and computer units, were installed at main neonatology/pediatric centers throughout the Tuscany region. Today, 13 hospitals are connected to the network, while the MEYER Pediatric University Hospital (MEYER) in Firenze has recently adhered to the project, as HUB center jointly with FTGM, so enabling H24 telemedicine service in pediatric cardiology throughout the region. So far, more than 200 patients were diagnosed and followed by telemedicine.

Keywords: telemedicine, tele-echocardiography, pediatric cardiology, congenital heart diseases

1. Introduction

In the last decades, the birth prevalence of congenital heart diseases progressively increased to a maximum of 9/1000 worldwide [1]. Echocardiography is the most commonly used noninvasive cardiovascular imaging modality and is considered to be both safe and cost-effective, but often expert evaluation of heart malformations is not usually available in community hospitals. Advancements in technology and broadband have allowed to set up effective tele-echocardiography services, now routinely used for transmitting cardiovascular ultrasound images to remote consultation centers for expert analysis and interpretation [2]. Thus, prompt accurate decision-making involving therapeutic or intervention planning is enabled, early in the fetus before delivery, in the newborn, or in the child up to adult patient.

The Gabriele Monasterio Tuscany Foundation (FTGM) (www.ftgm.it) is a healthcare institution of the public regional system, specialized in multidisciplinary research, diagnosis, and care of cardiovascular diseases, including interventional cardiology and cardiac surgery in both adult and pediatric patients. The FTGM Heart Hospital in Massa is currently a regional reference center for surgical and interventional treatment in neonatal and pediatric patients, as well as for fetal diagnosis of heart malformations. At FTGM the medical informatics staff has long time expertise in clinical information technology.

Ten years ago, the Pediatric Cardiology and Cardiac Surgery teams of the FTGM Heart Hospital in Massa, supported by the medical informatics researchers jointly with the volunteers of "Un Cuore un Mondo" Association, were involved in the International Healthcare Cooperation program of Tuscany region. The goal was to set up a cooperative network with the clinical centers in the Balkan countries, from Croatia to Bosnia-Herzegovina, Albania, and Romania, for supporting by telemedicine the diagnosis and care of congenital heart malformations.

Tele-echocardiography system was first implemented by the FTGM medical informatics staff at Pediatric Clinical Centers of Banja Luka (BIH) and Rijeka (KR), at the Gynecology Hospital in Tirana (AL). Later, other centers in Bosnia-Herzegovina (Gynecology Hospital in Sarajevo and Pediatric Hospitals in Tuzla and Mostar) as well as in Romania (Bucharest) were involved [3, 4]. Newborn and young patients with suspected heart malformations were evaluated on demand by tele-echocardiography from pediatric cardiologists at the HUB in Massa assessing the abnormal or critical cases. Up to 100 were transferred from Albania, Bosnia-Herzegovina, and Croatia for cardiac surgery. Each patient or fetus was first examined by tele-echocardiography in most of the cases. Even pregnant women, in case of critical fetal abnormalities, were transferred before delivery to the birth center in Massa to allow prompt intervention on newborns for limiting risks. Follow-up of patients, going back to home, was facilitated by the use of the telemedicine network.

Later, jointly with the National Research Council (CNR) Institute of Clinical Physiology (CNR-IFC), the FTGM participated to the European IPA Program in the project AdriHealthMob aimed at developing a cross-border model of services for healthcare in the Adriatic area. Fifteen partners of eight countries (Albania, Bosnia-Herzegovina, Croatia, Greece, Italy, Montenegro, Serbia, and Slovenia) were involved. AdriHealthMob platform for eHealth and eCare was designed for providing service through distance support for the rationalization of mobility up to the elimination of useless transfers for health and care [5, 6].

Four years ago, in Tuscany (a region in central Italy with 3 million of inhabitants, comprising a couple of major islands) the Lions Clubs achieved a grant (GA 14451/108-LA) from their International Foundation (LCIF) (www.lions.org) to support the FTGM for developing the regional telemedicine network in pediatric cardiology. This project (**Figure 1**) was launched in April 2015 with the aim of implementing pediatric tele-echocardiography for the diagnosis and care of cardiac malformations in neonatal and pediatric patients, as well as for follow-up of patients undergoing cardiac surgery. The main neonatology/pediatric hospital units throughout the Tuscany region were first interconnected with the pediatric cardiology department at FTGM Heart Hospital in Massa and later with MEYER Pediatric University Hospital (MEYER) in Firenze. Now, the FTGM and MEYER jointly serve as HUB reference center in the regional network, enabling H24 telemedicine service.

Tele-echocardiography is a process in which a provider or a technician obtains cardiovascular ultrasound images from a given patient, and these images are transmitted to an off-site location where a cardiologist can provide further analysis and interpretation. Thus, tele-echocardiography allows expert interpretation and consultation, promptly and without geographical limits, enabling accurate decision-making on triage, transport, and therapeutic or interventional plans [2].

Tele-echocardiography has been largely applied in pediatric cardiology over many years since the first live transmission of neonatal echocardiograms [7, 8]. The impact of telemedicine on delivery of pediatric cardiac care in community hospitals was assessed in many studies [9]. This approach was effective to increase

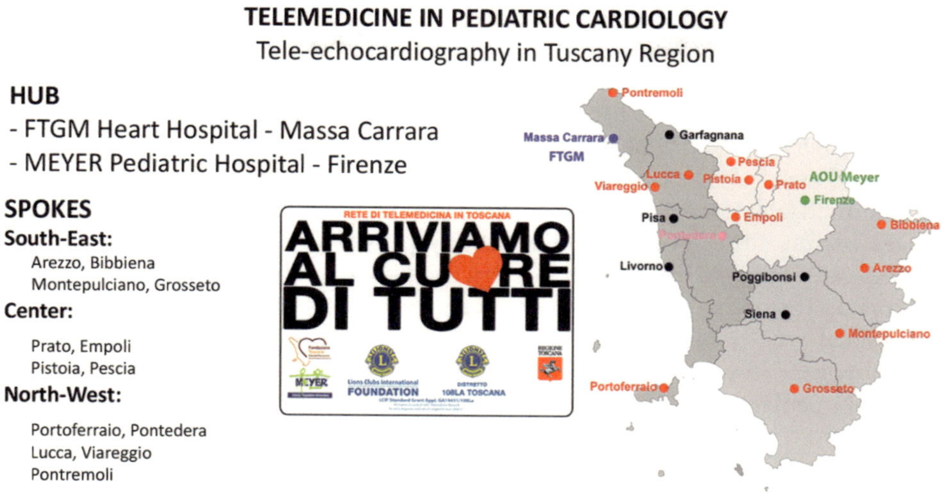

Figure 1.
Telemedicine network supported by lions clubs and their international foundation (LCIF) with the promotion of Tuscany region.

efficiency and quality of care, to improve echo examination quality, to prevent unnecessary transport of babies without critical heart disease, to enhance sonographer skill level, to yield financial savings, to decrease length of hospitalization, and to raise patient and physician satisfaction. More and more institutions are implementing tele-echocardiography [2, 10–18].

Basically, the physician ("operator"), observing the patient by echocardiography in community hospital, contacts the pediatric cardiologist at the reference center ("consultant") to obtain expert-enlightened joint diagnosis. In fact, while echography allows recognizing complex cardiac malformations, in neonate or even in fetus, often in community hospitals, the operator is not skilled to perform this analysis, and live guidance during patient examination is demanded to achieve actual diagnostic images. Thus, synchronous approach (online or live) in tele-echocardiography is preferred to the store-and-forward modality (recording echo-images and subsequently transmitting to the consultant).

2. Methods

HUB-and-SPOKE network was designed, interconnecting reference center of pediatric cardiology (HUB) with remote healthcare institution (SPOKE). Each SPOKE was securely connected to the HUB by encryption technology (VPN IPSec) through the institutional regional network (RTRT). Video communication technology was applied preferring hardware codec (coder-decoder) (H323 IP, download/upload >512 kbps) to software applications in order to enable friendly, effective, and reliable implementation, allowing to transmit echo-images in addition to videoconference signals [19]. The echo video signal is acquired from echography equipment, preferably through digital outputs (HDMI, DVI-D, display port), and transmitted by the codec to the consultant workstation. Standard compression (H264) is applied for allowing effective streaming and high diagnostic accuracy is assured in clinical practice, as reported in a number of studies [20, 21].

This solution was first applied for implementing tele-echocardiography in Balkan countries and later in the Tuscany region, where the FTGM and MEYER pediatric cardiology staff jointly served as HUB consultant center.

Live tele-echocardiography was implemented by the use of codecs at the two sides of the network (SPOKE and HUB), streaming echo-images over network from the echography room of community hospital to the consultant center during videoconference. Store-and-forward facility was provided to allow transmission of full-resolution DICOM images from echography equipment to HUB server for revision of live evaluation or off-line second-opinion evaluation. This option was also useful to overcome possible drawbacks in synchronous transmission of echo-images, mainly due to performance instability of public networks.

The use of medical information system (internally developed in the FTGM by informatics researchers) allowed the operator to document patient medical history and clinical conditions, to record echocardiography findings, to print out disclosure and informed consent, and to record diagnostic evaluation in agreement with the consultant pediatric cardiologist (**Figure 2**). Actually, the final report is signed by

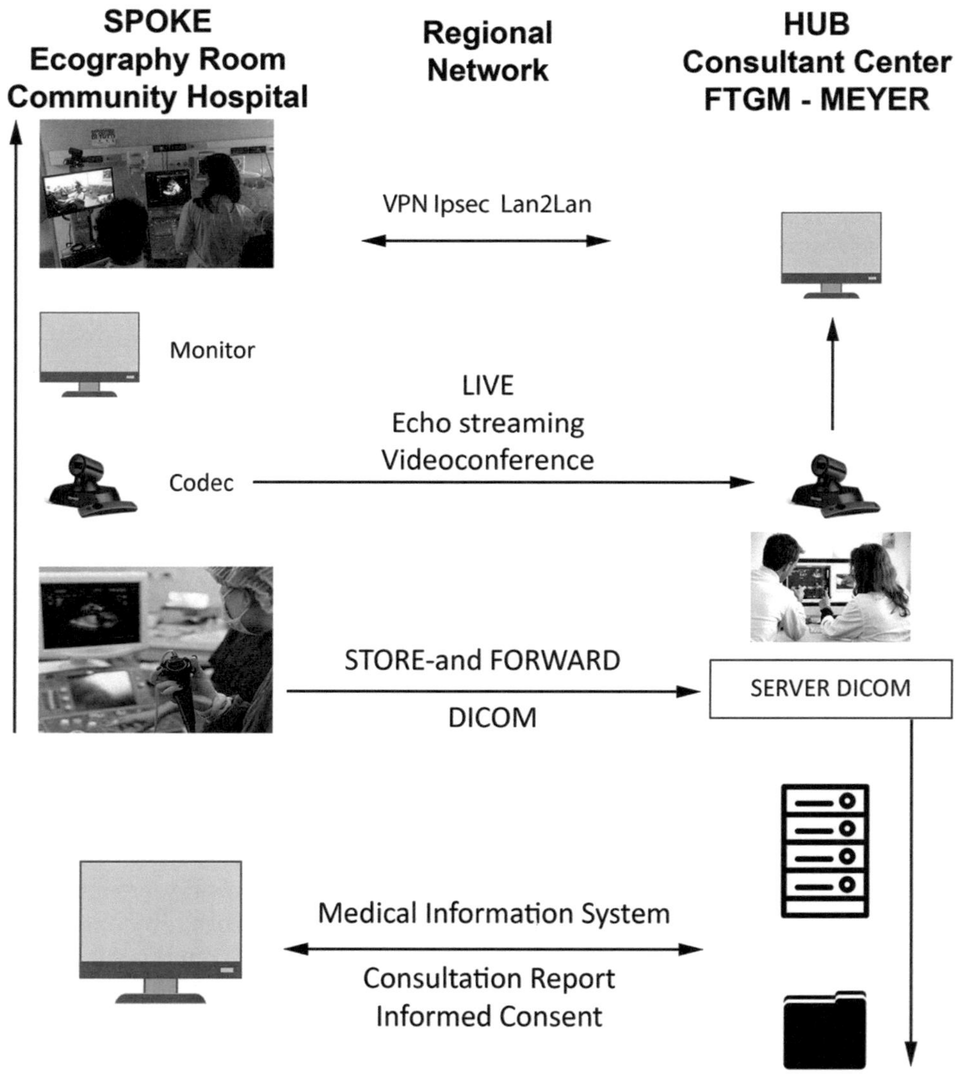

Figure 2.
Videoconference equipment was applied to implement live tele-echocardiography by secure connection of SPOKE setting with HUB center. DICOM images are transferred for revision and second opinion. Information system facilities are made available to manage diagnostic report and patient consent.

both the two physicians (the operator and the consultant) cooperating by telemedicine in patient diagnostic evaluation.

Tele-echocardiography session is a two-step process:

- First, live tele-echocardiography is achieved streaming echo-images during videoconference, so allowing the consultant to guide the operator for proper scanning of cardiac anatomy.

- Secondly, at the end of the patient echography examination, selected high-resolution DICOM images are transferred to the HUB center for allowing revision/confirmation of live diagnostic evaluations and definitive reporting.

Telemedicine guidelines, promoted in Italy by National Health System [22], were applied to set up regular and effective services for pediatric cardiology.

3. Regional telemedicine network in pediatric cardiology

Neonatology/pediatric units in Tuscany region are usually referred for diagnosis and care of cardiac malformations to two reference institutions: the FTGM Heart Hospital in Massa and the MEYER Pediatric University Hospital in Firenze.

Considering the great number (thousands each year) of outpatient visits at both FTGM and MEYER hospitals, telemedicine technology has a potential impact on healthcare throughout the region, facilitating expert evaluation and follow-up of so many patients. Families of young patients will benefit too, avoiding traveling with physical and emotional burden while saving money but also achieving early treatment for better patient care.

Following previous experiences in Balkan countries, FTGM developed the project "Arriviamo al Cuore di Tutti" to set up a pediatric tele-echocardiography network in Tuscany, aimed at interconnecting the reference centers (initially FTGM Heart Hospital in Massa and recently MEYER in Firenze) with main clinical centers throughout the region.

The Public Department of Health of the Region of Tuscany promoted the development of telemedicine network in pediatric cardiology, while the Lions Clubs of Tuscany (District 108LA), jointly with their International Foundation, contributed financial support to purchase all equipment for implementing teleconsultation service (**Figure 2**) [6].

According to telemedicine guidelines, promoted in Italy by the National Health System [22], the main goal was to allow accurate decision-making on the basis of the collaborative interaction between the echocardiography operator at each SPOKE and the expert pediatric cardiologist at the HUB (FTGM and MEYER).

Management and technical assistance are due to the FTGM technical staff and the technical organization of regional healthcare institutions (ESTAR).

Neonatology, cardiology, or pediatric care units of remote hospital (SPOKE) were provided with telemedicine workstations, able to transmit echocardiography images during the videoconference session, each one securely interconnected with the specialist center (HUB), serving teleconsultation or second-opinion requests. The HUB, facilities were provided for allowing multicenter videoconference, exchanging clinical data, and recording DICOM echocardiography images (**Figure 2**).

VPN communication infrastructure suitable for assuring, by standard IPSec protocol, security, and protection of health data, was set up over the existing regional large bandwidth infrastructure, interconnecting public institutions in Tuscany, by the FTGM medical informatics staff in collaboration with their colleagues of the regional technical organization. The tele-echocardiography workstations were installed by FTGM staff at each SPOKE taking into account local needs or preferences of healthcare personnel.

Particular attention was dedicated to the training aspects for allowing effective at-distance collaboration in echocardiography evaluation of cardiac malformations. Initially, the training of SPOKE healthcare staff was planned at the Heart Hospital pediatric department or at their departments, while videoconferencing interaction during tele-echocardiography allowed the operator physicians to improve at distance more and more their skill throughout the project. Guides for management and troubleshooting of telemedicine service were provided by FTGM.

Consultation or second-opinion sessions were initially scheduled, involving pediatric cardiology staff at FTGM, with the assistance of computer technicians, while 24/7 regular service is being organized for management of emergency, urgent, and elective cases.

Live tele-echocardiography (as described in Methods) was implemented using videoconferencing equipment (codec), able to capture echo-images from ultrasound signal and to transmit them from the SPOKE over the network to the HUB by efficient standard compression (H264). So, the echo-images, examined by the operator at SPOKE center, are simultaneously replicated on the monitor at the HUB center (FTGM) where the pediatric cardiologist (the consultant), by videoconferencing interaction, is allowed to help the colleague achieving correct heart examination so cooperating to diagnostic evaluation.

The codec (Lifesize ICON 400), the monitor, and the video-camera were mounted on a mobile cart equipped with medical insulators on each external connection (ultrasound, network, and power lines) to allow movement and safe use in the hospital settings. The so-equipped system allows the consultant from the HUB to express a diagnostic opinion, so contributing to define one report, shared with the patient doctor at the SPOKE center. The telemedicine cart included a compact-type computer for medical reporting and optionally a printer (**Figures 3** and **4**).

Echography equipment was configured to allow (at the end of the examination) the transmission of selected heart images in DICOM format to the HUB server (store-and-forward option). These native resolution images allowed revision and confirmation of the "live" diagnostic evaluation. Moreover, this "off-line" modality will be useful for backup in case of connection failures or quality degradation during live session.

At each SPOKE center, a medical record application, developed and adapted by FTGM informatics staff, was made available [5]. Disclosure and informed consent (**Figure 5**) is recorded according to the privacy rules. Patient information is entered into the medical record (anamnesis, physical examination, diagnostic reports, conclusions); final report is achieved including signatures of both the operator and the consultant. New web-based release has been recently introduced to facilitate medical reporting.

Connection between the two HUB centers (FTGM and MEYER) also allows joint clinical discussion by videoconference, sharing all information on patients, particularly useful in the evaluation of complex and critical cases.

The physician at SPOKE center (operator) calls the HUB center (FTGM or MEYER) for activating videoconference connection and opens the medical record at the HUB to document patient history and physical examination. The informed consent is printed out and signed by the young patient's parents. The patient is identified on ultrasound equipment for allowing DICOM transmission at the end of the examination.

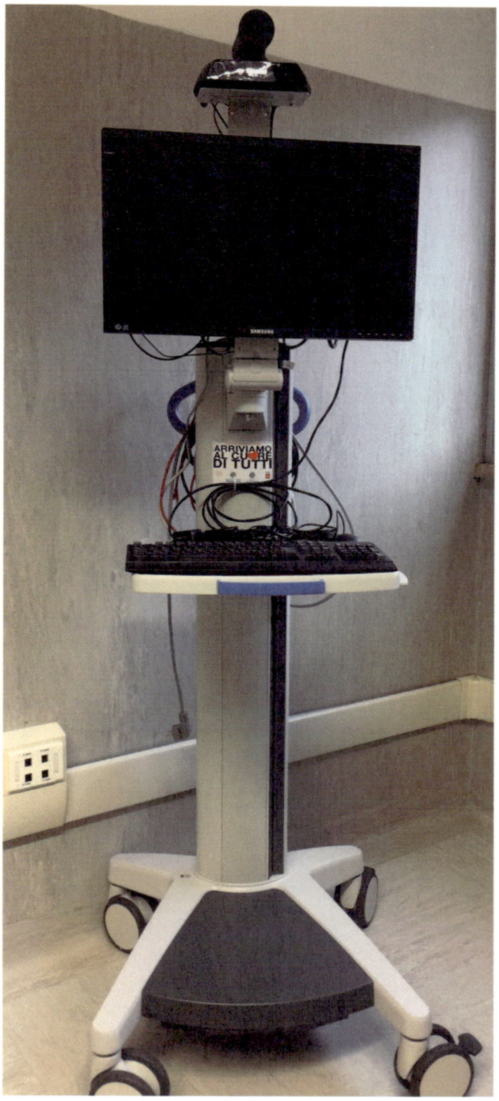

Figure 3.
Mobile medical-grade cart, equipped with videoconferencing and computer workstation, allowing use in clinical setting.

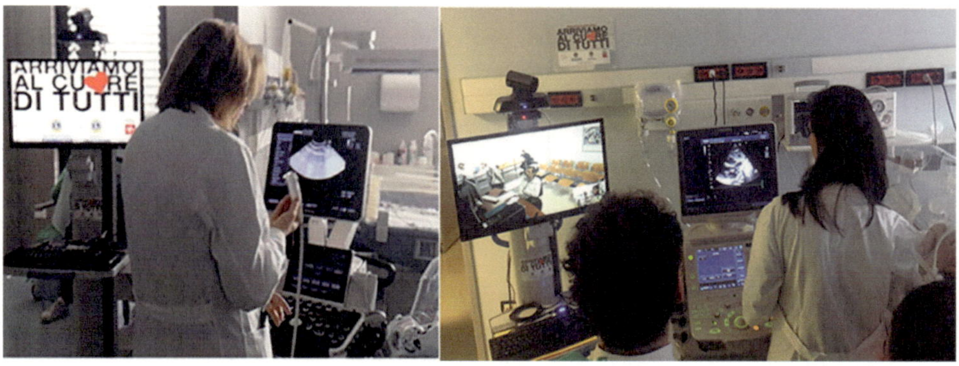

Figure 4.
Tele-echocardiography from neonatology (Prato and Viareggio).

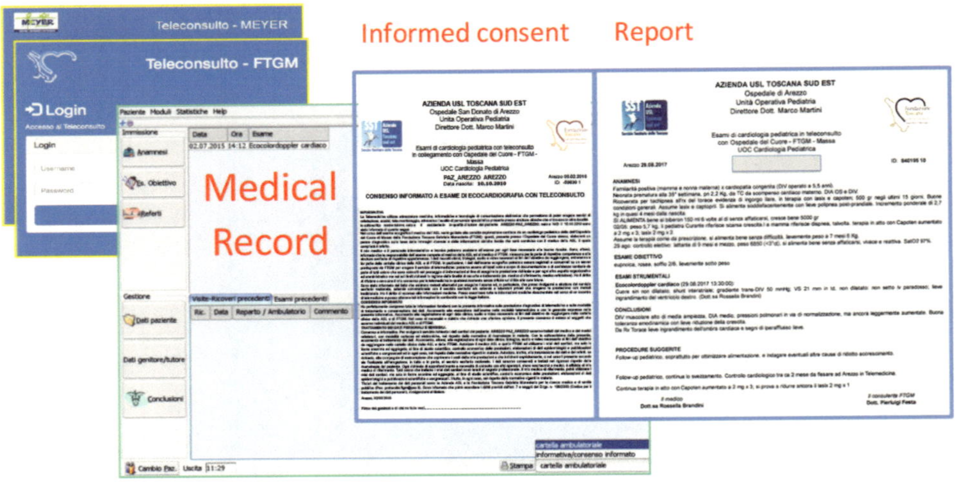

Figure 5.
The patient medical record, accessed by the user's password in the HUB/SPOKE network, is applied for documentation and for echocardiography reporting.

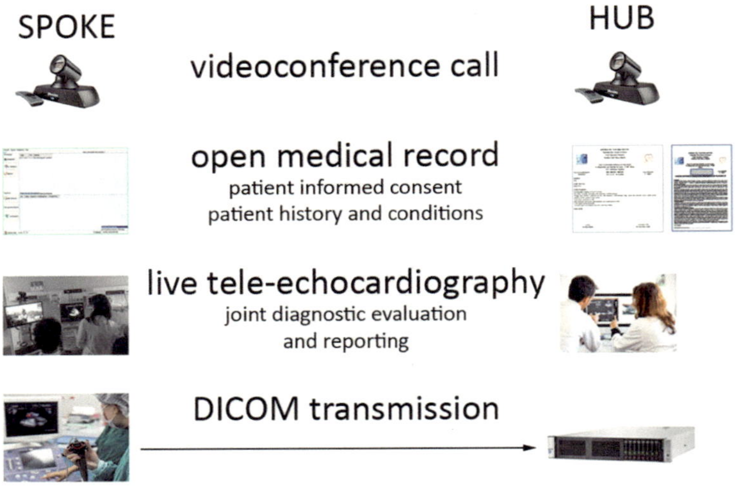

Figure 6.
Main steps of tele-echocardiography session.

Tele-echocardiography session starts with videoconference interaction between the operator and consultant: ultrasound images are "live" replicated at the HUB workstation for allowing cooperation of the consultant to diagnostic evaluation (**Figure 6**).

3.1 Research objectives

The aim of this project was to develop a telemedicine network for supporting medical decision-making in pediatric cardiology throughout the region, particularly in the diagnosis and care of heart malformations, usually referring to few specialized institutions. Large distances separate the patient and nonspecialist from expert advice.

Videoconference technology and medical information system solutions, previously internally developed in FTGM, were applied and implemented to set up a regional network, interconnecting HUB institutions (FTGM and MEYER Hospitals) with neonatology, pediatrics, cardiology, or gynecology (SPOKE) centers. Each SPOKE center was equipped with tele-echocardiography workstation, allowing "live" consultation/second opinion in addition to face-to-face interaction for clinical discussion and care planning; medical record system was implemented for patient data exchange and reporting, and store-and-forward DICOM facility was provided for revision and documentation.

The main research objectives are summarized as follows:

- Set up low-cost/effective telemedicine network for supporting medical decision-making in pediatric cardiology.
- Allow collaborative medical decision-making for improving overall quality of care and promoting a real clinical network.
- Healthcare cost reduction avoiding unnecessary patient transfers or hospitalizations.

4. Results

Initially, the hospital of Elba island, in the south part of Tuscany, was involved as a pilot SPOKE center: secure network connection (VPN IPSec) was set up with the Heart Hospital in Massa (183 Km far away plus one hour for ship travel); the video output of the ultrasound equipment was connected to videoconference codec for streaming images to the HUB (**Figure 2**).

After the pilot action in Elba island, tele-echocardiography service was progressively deployed in all the provinces throughout the Tuscany region.

List of active SPOKE centers:

1. Elba island hospital (pediatrics)
2. Lucca (outpatient cardiology)
3. Empoli (outpatient cardiology)
4. Pontremoli (internal medicine)
5. Arezzo (ICU neonatology/pediatrics, outpatient cardiology)
6. Bibbiena (outpatient cardiology unit)
7. Prato (ICU neonatology and outpatient cardiology) (**Figure 4**)
8. Montepulciano (ICU neonatology/pediatrics, outpatient cardiology)
9. Viareggio (ICU neonatology/pediatrics department) (**Figure 4**)
10. Pistoia (pediatrics and cardiology)
11. Pescia (outpatient cardiology)
12. Pontedera (outpatient cardiology)
13. Grosseto (outpatient cardiology)

Another center was recently connected out of the region: Hospital of Cagliari (Sardinia region) (ICU neonatology/pediatrics).

According to the functional layout of **Figure 6**, "live" tele-echocardiography session is followed by "off-line" transmission of DICOM records to FTGM server for revision, while medical record system (running on FTGM server) is made available at the SPOKE center for documenting clinical conditions and for recording the report, agreed by both the physician operator at SPOKE and the specialist consultant at HUB. Information disclosure and informed consent are provided in agreement with legal constraints.

H24 tele-echocardiography service will be organized, jointly by the two HUB centers (FTGM and MEYER), to enable management of both urgent and elective cases.

SPOKE centers have started gradually their telemedicine activity: up to 200 patients (300 visits) were so far examined by tele-echocardiography.

The most active center resulted the pediatric department at Arezzo Hospital.

4.1 Telemedicine from Arezzo hospital

From April 2016 to May 2018, at the pediatric department of Arezzo Hospital, 65 live tele-echocardiography sessions in connection with the FTGM HUB have been performed in 26 children (from newborn until 6-year ones). Reports were produced by medical record system and DICOM images were also transmitted for revision and documentation. In 22 children (84.6%), telemedicine session was electively scheduled, whereas in 4 children, urgent remote specialized advice was required. The most frequent indication was heart murmur in 10, cyanosis in 9, and poor growth in 7 children. Only in one case, tele-echocardiography was inadequate for complete diagnosis. The most frequent diagnosis was the perimembranous ventricular defect (13/26, 50%), followed by atrial septum defect (2), partial pulmonary venous return (2), AV canal (2), hypoplastic aortic arch (1), pulmonary stenosis (1), and hypertrophic cardiomyopathy (1). Only in one case, echocardiography examination resulted completely normal.

Four telemedicine consultations were carried out in emergency: one patient was transferred for urgent surgical intervention (AV canal), two patients were electively operated after medical therapy bridge (hypertrophic cardiomyopathy and perimembranous ventricular septal defect), and the last one initiated optimal medical therapy for dilated cardiomyopathy. Twenty-two children were scheduled for elective follow-up: 1 after surgery and 21 before surgery. Seven outpatients underwent surgery: two for atrial septum defect OS, two for partial pulmonary venous return, three for perimembranous ventricular defect. Of the remaining 14 children, seven were followed up by telemedicine, and for the other ones normal follow-up was preferred. Therefore, unnecessary transfer to the regional HUB unit was avoided in 15 out of 26 patients.

5. Conclusions

Heart malformations in infants are very serious because they can affect the child's life if not cared from the very first hours after birth. The FTGM Heart Hospital is highly specialized in pediatric cardiac surgery, which annually saves many children coming from Italy and abroad, even from disadvantaged countries outside Europe.

In 2015 by the cooperation between the medical and technical professionals at FTGM, the telemedicine project in diagnosis and care of cardiac malformations ("Arriviamo al Cuore di Tutti") was launched with financial support provided from both the Lions Clubs of Tuscany (district 108La) and the Lions Clubs International Foundation. The regional public health system approved this initiative promoting collaboration between healthcare institutions throughout the region.

Lions/LCIF budget enabled to purchase medical and computer equipment at the SPOKE hospitals in addition to server facilities at HUB center at both FTGM and MEYER.

Tele-echocardiography allowed collaborative medical decision-making in diagnosis and care of complex and critical heart defects. It played an important role in the early diagnosis, follow-up, or exclusion of cardiovascular abnormalities, planning patient mobility to tertiary specialist center when really necessary [23].

Now, 13 tele-echocardiography workstations have been installed in Tuscany and another one in Sardinia.

We expect that regional health authorities will continue to promote telemedicine service, dealing with reimbursement aspects and monitoring activity in the next years. Assistance and maintenance support will be likely organized in collaboration with the regional technical staff.

The main benefits of telemedicine network are summarized:

- Shortening the time to diagnosis limiting risks for patient
- Preventing unnecessary patient transports and avoiding discomforts for families
- Promoting a real clinical network, fostering collaboration between physicians and empowering the medical skill out of all centers
- Extending specialized remote consultation for follow-up of patients undergoing high-specialty interventions
- Improving quality of care in pediatric cardiology
- Reducing costs for both families and the public health system

As previously reported (Section 4.1) according to the experience at Arezzo Hospital, the effectiveness of the telemedicine network was assessed, while further developments are expected as more centers become really active. Transfers of newborns/children were avoided in many cases (58% in Arezzo) when could be good managed in place avoiding, consequently, unnecessary costs and patient/family discomforts. Inappropriate transfers to intermediate neonatal cardiology units have been also avoided, referring the baby directly to the regional cardiac surgery service at FTGM HUB, when necessary. Finally, telemedicine allowed pediatric cardiologists at SPOKE centers to improve their skill through the interaction with experienced and specialized colleagues at HUB center.

The main drawback, limiting the full application of the network, depends on the training needed for using new technology but also on the willingness of operators to dedicate extra time, at least initially, for telemedicine-based examination.

The extension of use of tele-echocardiography in fetal diagnosis of cardiac malformations would allow early diagnosis for planning care and interventions already at delivery time at the specialized center. Moreover, the telemedicine network, now focused on pediatric cardiology, could be extended to other medical pathologies, also in adults just providing remote specialized medical care around the region [24–29].

Advances in information technology and lower costs allow telemedicine empowerment according to the needs of physicians also outside the hospital setting.

Acknowledgements

Thanks to Lions Clubs of the District 108La (Tuscany) and to the Lions Clubs International Foundation (LCIF) for financially supporting this project, particularly to Dr. Gianluca Rocchi, Lions District 108La Governor in 2014/2015, for promoting and supporting the implementation of the network.

We thank for collaborative effort both clinical, technical, and administrative teams of clinical centers participating to this project; the list of the main collaborators (clinical, technical) is as follows: Elba Hospital (Bruno Graziano, Duilio Biani and Alberto Iurato, Marco Galletti), Lucca (Andrea Azzarelli, Riccardo Orsini), Empoli (Anna Monopoli), Pontremoli (Mauro Cozzalupi, Renzo Bresciani), Arezzo (Marco Martini and Rossella Brandini, Maurizio Pasquini), Bibbiena (Moreno Marri), Montepulciano (Jessica Attene), Prato (Pierluigi Vasarri and Anna Maria Traini, Fabio Noferi), Pistoia (Michela Taglioli), Pescia (Stefano Di Marco), Pontedera (Laura Papi), Grosseto (Alberto Cresti), and Viareggio (Elisa Ferrali).

Special thanks to the pediatric cardiology staff at MEYER Pediatric Hospital (Silvia Favilli; Marco Curradi), recently involved in the project.

Finally, thanks to the FTGM staff (clinical, technical, and administrative), particularly to Giuseppe Santoro (pediatric cardiology), Bruno Murzi (pediatric cardiac surgery), and Medical Informatics collaborators in Massa e Pisa (Maurizio Mangione, Gianna Alberini, Mario Cossu, Mauro Micalizzi, Giacomo Piccini, Emiliano Rocca, Tiziano Carducci, Andrea Gori, and colleagues).

Conflict of interest

The authors declare no conflict of interest.

Funding

This project ("Arriviamo al Cuore di Tutti") was jointly financed by Lions Clubs of Tuscany region and the Lions Clubs International Foundation (LCIF, www.lcif.org), under the promotion of regional healthcare authorities. A grant of 71.000 US$ (GA 14451/108-LA) was provided from the LCIF in 2015, in addition to the contribution of local Clubs, up to a total project budget of 170.000 euro.

The FTGM, supported by the Lions Clubs and LCIF and promoted by regional authorities, contacted the main healthcare institutions throughout Tuscany for planning implementation of tele-echocardiography service. Formal agreements were set up for experimentation defining legal issues for care delivery cooperation in pediatric cardiology. The regional technical healthcare organization (ESTAR) was contacted for scheduling, in collaboration with FTGM informatics staff, VPN networking, and installation of workstations at SPOKE centers.

The financial budget, provided by Lions/LCIF, was sufficient to purchase hardware and software for implementing telemedicine workstations in each SPOKE, while technicians from both FTGM and the regional health system organization jointly contributed to set up the HUB-and-SPOKE VPN network.

Author details

Alessandro Taddei[1,2*], Pierluigi Festa[1], Fabrizio Conforti[1], Giuseppe Santoro[1], Gianluca Rocchi[2] and Luciano Ciucci[1,2,3]

1 Gabriele Monasterio Tuscany Foundation, Heart Hospital, Massa, Italy

2 Lions Clubs International, Tuscany, Italy

3 Gabriele Monasterio Tuscany Foundation, Pisa, Italy

*Address all correspondence to: alessandro.taddei@ftgm.it

IntechOpen

© 2019 The Author(s). Licensee IntechOpen. This chapter is distributed under the terms of the Creative Commons Attribution License (http://creativecommons.org/licenses/by/3.0), which permits unrestricted use, distribution, and reproduction in any medium, provided the original work is properly cited.

References

[1] Liu Y, Chen S, Zühlke L, Black GC, Choy M, Li N, et al. Global birth prevalence of congenital heart defects 1970-2017: Updated systematic review and meta-analysis of 260 studies. International Journal of Epidemiology. 2019;**48**(2):455-463. DOI: 10.1093/ije/dyz009

[2] Satou GM, Rheuban K, Alverson D, Lewin M, Mahnke C, Marcin J, et al. Telemedicine in pediatric cardiology: A scientific statement from the American Heart Association. Circulation. 2017;**135**:e648-e678. DOI: 10.1161/CIR.0000000000000478

[3] Taddei A, Dalmiani S, Vellani A, Rocca E, Piccini G, Carducci T, et al. Data integration in cardiac surgery health care institution: Experience at G. Pasquinucci heart hospital. In: Proceedings of Computers in Cardiology; 14-17 September 2008; Bologna: IEEE. 2008. pp. 287-290. DOI: 10.1109/CIC.2008.4749034

[4] Taddei A, Gori A, Rocca E, Carducci T, Piccini G, Augiero G, et al. Telemedicine network for early diagnosis and care of heart malformations. In: Zhang YT, editor. The International Conference on Health Informatics. IFMBE Proceedings. Vol. 42. Cham: Springer; 2014. pp. 268-271. DOI: 10.1007/978-3-319-03005-0_68

[5] Taddei A, Gori A, Rocca E, Carducci T, Piccini G, Augiero G, et al. Telemedicine in collaborative diagnosis and care of congenital heart malformations. In: Rinaldi G, editor. New Perspectives in Medical Records. TELe-Health. Cham: Springer; 2017. pp. 185-197. DOI: 10.1007/978-3-319-28661-7_16

[6] Taddei A, Augiero G, Ciregia A, Conforti F, Cossu M, Gori A, et al. Regional telemedicine network for diagnosis and care of cardiac malformations. In: Berhardt LV, editor. Advances in Medicine and Biology. Vol. 116. New York: Nova Science Publishers; 2017. pp. 21-45

[7] Casey F, Brown D, Craig BG, Rogers J, Mulholland HC. Diagnosis of neonatal congenital heart defects by remote consultation using a low-cost telemedicine link. Journal of Telemedicine and Telecare. 1996;**2**:165-169. DOI: 10.1258/1357633961930004

[8] Sable CA, Cummings SD, Pearson GD, Schratz LM, Cross RC, Quivers ES, et al. Impact of telemedicine on the practice of pediatric cardiology in community hospitals. Pediatrics. 2002;**109**(1):e3-e3. DOI: 10.1542/peds.109.1.e3

[9] Krishnan A, Fuska M, Dixon R, Sable CA. The evolution of pediatric tele-echocardiography: 15-year experience of over 10,000 transmissions. Telemedicine Journal and E-Health. 2014;**20**(8):681-686. DOI: 10.1089/tmj.2013.0279

[10] Adambounou K, Adjenou V, Salam AP, Farin F, N'Dakena KG, Gbeassor M, et al. A low-cost tele-imaging platform for developing countries. Frontiers in Public Health. 2014;**2**:135. DOI: 10.3389/fpubh.2014.00135

[11] Grant B, Morgan GJ, McCrossan BA, Crealey GE, Sands AJ, Craig B, et al. Remote diagnosis of congenital heart disease: The impact of telemedicine. Archives of Disease in Childhood. 2010;**95**(4):276-280. DOI: 10.1136/adc.2008.146456

[12] Mars M. Telemedicine and advances in urban and rural healthcare delivery in Africa. Progress in Cardiovascular Diseases. 2013;**56**(3):326-335. DOI: 10.1016/j.pcad.2013.10.006

[13] McCrossan BA, Doherty NN, Sands AJ, Grant B, Craig BG, McCusker CG, et al. Survey of paediatricians' opinions on a regional paediatric telecardiology service. Journal of Paediatrics and Child Health. 2014;**50**(6):482-486. DOI: 10.1111/jpc.12501

[14] Singh S, Bansal M, Maheshwari P, Adams D, Sengupta SP, Price R, et al. American society of echocardiography: Remote echocardiography with web-based assessments for referrals at a distance (ASE-REWARD) study. Journal of the American Society of Echocardiography. 2013;**26**(3):221-233. DOI: 10.1016/j.echo.2012.12.012

[15] Sasangohar F, Davis E, Kash BA, Shah SR. Remote patient monitoring and telemedicine in neonatal and pediatric settings: Scoping literature review. Journal of Medical Internet Research. 2018;**20**(12):e295. DOI: 10.2196/jmir.9403

[16] Maia MR, Castela E, Pires A, Lapão LV. How to develop a sustainable telemedicine service? A Pediatric Telecardiology Service 20 years on—An exploratory study. BMC Health Services Research. 2019;**19**:681. DOI: 10.1186/s12913-019-4511-5

[17] Pick JM, Watson R, Lee I, Lee B, Gearhart A, Batra AS. The feasibility of telemedicine in pediatric cardiology. Journal of Pediatrics & Neonatal Care. 2018;**8**(3):121-124. DOI: 10.15406/jpnc.2018.08.00322

[18] Rouse CA, Woods BT, Mahnke CB. A retrospective analysis of a pediatric tele-echocardiography service to treat, triage, and reduce trans-Pacific transport. Journal of Telemedicine and Telecare. 2018;**24**(3):224-229. DOI: 10.1177/1357633X16689500

[19] Liu W, Zhan K, Locatis C, Ackerman M. Internet-based videoconferencing coder/decoders and tools for telemedicine. Telemedicine Journal and E-Health. 2011;**17**(5):358-362. DOI: 10.1089/tmj.2010.0193

[20] Lewin M, Xu C, Jordan M, Borchers H, Ayton C, Wilbert D, et al. Accuracy of paediatric echocardiographic transmission via telemedicine. Journal of Telemedicine and Telecare. 2006;**12**(8):416-421

[21] Barbier P, Dalla Vecchia L, Mirra G, Di Marco S, Cavoretto D. Near real-time echocardiography teleconsultation using low bandwidth and MPEG-4 compression: Feasibility, image adequacy and clinical implications. Journal of Telemedicine and Telecare. 2012;**18**(4):204-210

[22] Italian Ministry of Health. National Telemedicine Guidelines. 2014. Available from: http://www.salute.gov.it/imgs/C_17_pubblicazioni_2129_allegato.pdf [Accessed: 2019-10-03]

[23] Otto CA, Shemenski R, Drudi L. Real-time tele-echocardiography: Diagnosis and management of a pericardial effusion secondary to pericarditis at an Antarctic research station. Telemedicine Journal and E-Health. 2012;**18**(7):521-524. DOI: 10.1089/tmj.2011.0266

[24] Raikhelkar J, Raikhelkar JK. The impact of telemedicine in cardiac critical care. Critical Care Clinics. 2015;**31**(2):305-317. DOI: 10.1016/j.ccc.2014.12.008

[25] Murni IK, Musa NL. The need for specialized pediatric cardiac critical care training program in limited resource settings. Frontiers in Pediatrics. 2018;**6**:59. DOI: 10.3389/fped.2018.00059

[26] Hoffman AM, Lapcharoensap W, Trang Huynh T, Lund K. Historical perspectives: Telemedicine in neonatology. NeoReviews. 2019;**20**(3):e113-e123. DOI: 10.1542/neo.20-3-e113

[27] Latifi R, Parsikia A, Boci A, Doarn CR, Merrell RC. Increases access to care through telemedicine in Albania: An analysis of 2,724 patients. Telemedicine and e-Health. 2019. DOI: 10.1089/tmj.2018.0338. [Epub ahead of print]

[28] Raikhelkar J, Raikhelkar JK. Advances in tele-cardiology. In: Koenig M, editor. Telemedicine in the ICU. Cham: Springer; 2019. pp. 225-242. DOI: 10.1007/978-3-030-11569-2_13

[29] Muhsen W. An ECHO on the go: A case report on the importance of echocardiographic assessment skills in acute neonatal transport settings. Annales de Pédiatrie. 2019;**2**(1):1015

Section 2

Clinical Decision Support Systems (CDSS)

Chapter 5

Owning Attention: Applying Human Factors Principles to Support Clinical Decision Support

Robin Littlejohn, Ronald Romero Barrientos, Christian Boxley and Kristen Miller

Abstract

In the best examples, clinical decision support (CDS) systems guide clinician decision-making and actions, prevent errors, improve quality, reduce costs, save time, and promote the use of evidence-based recommendations. However, the potential solution that CDS represents are limited by problems associated with improper design, implementation, and local customization. Despite an emphasis on electronic health record usability, little progress has been made to protect end-users from inadequately designed workflows and unnecessary interruptions. Intelligent and personalized design creates an opportunity to tailor CDS not just at the patient level but specific to the disease condition, provider experience, and available resources at the healthcare system level. This chapter leverages the Five Rights of CDS framework to demonstrate the application of human factors engineering principles and emerging trends to optimize data analytics, usability, workflow, and design.

Keywords: clinical decision support, CDS Five Rights, electronic health record, human factors engineering, user-centered design

1. Current state of clinical decision support

Clinical decision support (CDS), leveraging features within the electronic health record (EHR), is increasingly recognized as a valuable tool for providing cognitive support for diagnosis, severity assessment, clinical management, and disposition. CDS is defined as "providing clinicians with clinical knowledge and patient-related information, intelligently filtered, and presented at appropriate times to enhance patient care" [1, 2]. In the best examples, CDS systems guide clinician decision-making and actions [3], prevent errors [4, 5], improve quality [6, 7], reduce costs [8], save time [9], and promote the use of evidence-based recommendations [10]. CDS has the potential to enable clinicians to better address rising information needs, providing the opportunity to pick up on subtle early indications of risk or vulnerability while sorting through an avalanche of data. The availability of evidence-based guidelines for clinical care and for CDS implementation encourages providers to deliver the best, evidence-based care available.

The potential solution that CDS represents is limited by problems associated with improper design, implementation, and local customization. The interaction of poorly designed technologies, organizational constraints, and lowered functional capability has the potential to multiply latent risks in healthcare technologies. Computerized systems that are designed to help clinicians make decisions fail two-thirds of the time as a result of factors such as providing incorrect information or providing information at a point that is incompatible with the workflow [11]. There are surprisingly low acceptance rates for some forms of CDS; approximately 91% of real-time CDS is overridden or ignored by clinicians due to time constraints, perceived misleading alerts, or their patients did not meet certain criteria (such as age or condition) [12]. High rates of alert overrides have been widely acknowledged as a deterrent to acceptance and appropriate use of CDS [13]. Alert overload is detrimental to clinician performance, not only because it can lead to errors by overriding true positive alerts, but also because the false alerts consume clinicians' time and mental resources. The overabundance of pop-ups, notifications, and check-boxes is highly distracting and produces sensory overload and a perception of extra work without value which contributes to the development of negative perceptions of health information technology. These negative perceptions contribute to low job satisfaction, early retirement, and high turnover [14]. As a result, research indicates that the use of automated, and real-time alerts are only modestly effective in increasing the performance of key tasks [15].

Backed by sophisticated analytics and algorithms to advance clinical decision-making, coupled with increasing pressure to increase throughput and reduce costs, the EHR is often thought to be the solution to the deadly problems of adverse events and inappropriate prescribing. However, the EHR often provides alerts that are perceived by the physicians as unnecessary and clinically insignificant, contributing to alert fatigue and provider burnout [16]. Despite an emphasis on EHR usability, little progress has been made to protect end-users from inadequately designed workflows and unnecessary interruptions [17]. Clinicians' lack of motivation to use CDS appears to be related to the perceived value of the function combined with the lack of integration into workflow [18]. By identifying factors that predict clinically insignificant alerts and inappropriate responses, informatics personnel can improve alert logic to account for factors such as workflow and patient complexity, increasing specificity of alerts. As a result of the improved specificity, clinicians may experience less alert fatigue, override fewer alerts, and provide better care for patients with conditions that warrant serious alerts. The ultimate goal is to integrate clinical research with human factors engineering to develop optimized CDS systems to satisfy the information needs of clinicians as they formulate, debate, and discuss next steps in treatment or diagnostics for patients. CDS interventions improve care processes and outcomes when they achieve the CDS Five Rights—i.e., deliver the right information to the right people using the right formats via the right channels at the right times in the workflow [19]. This chapter leverages the Five Rights of CDS framework to describe good and bad examples of CDS design, development, and implementation; demonstrate the application of human factors engineering principles to CDS; and describe emerging trends to optimize data analytics, usability, workflow, and design.

2. Application of human factors engineering

Human factors engineering (HFE) is an established scientific discipline used in many high-reliability organizations. HFE takes a system approach to identify crucial components of the man-machine interface and human interactions such as communication, teamwork, and culture. By acknowledging human limitations and system vulnerabilities, HFE minimizes and mitigates human frailties to optimize system performance [20]. Given the complexity of healthcare systems and processes, current HFE healthcare research emphasizes the need for increasing partnerships between human factors engineers and clinical medicine to enhance the standard of care through in-depth evaluation and thoughtful system redesign. Human factors principles, standards, and guidelines provide considerations for the design and development of CDS.

Human factors principles suggest that the format and presentation of the CDS may not be readily applied in the busy acute clinical setting and fail to provide confidence to clinical staff. Effective presentation of an alert, including how and what is displayed, may offer better cognitive support during busy patient encounters and may help providers extract information quickly. Following good human factors principles, alerts should signal to an important matter, inform, and guide the provider [21]. Traditionally, alerts are system components that serve to direct a user's attention to information related to a value that has exceeded a parameter threshold [22]. Newer alerts, however, have advanced to the point of becoming a "type of automation that supplements the human powers of observation and decision" [23]. Alerts amplify the capacity of clinicians to continuously monitor changes in patient status and thereby support timely intervention. Alerts should be prioritized according to the severity of consequence that could be prevented by taking corrective action (severity) and according to the time available for successful corrective action to be performed (urgency). Substantial human factors analysis remains to be done to realize the potential benefits of CDS.

3. Five Rights of CDS

A useful framework for achieving success in CDS design, development, and implementation is the "CDS Five Rights" approach [24]. The CDS Five Rights model states that we can achieve CDS-supported improvements in desired healthcare outcomes if we communicate: [1] the right information: evidence-based, suitable to guide action, pertinent to the circumstance; [2] to the right person: considering all members of the care team, including clinicians, patients, and their caretakers; [3] in the right CDS intervention format: such as an alert, order set, or reference information to answer a clinical question; [4] through the right channel: for example, a clinical information system such as the EHR, a personal health record (PHR), or a more general channel such as the Internet or a mobile device; [5] at the right time in workflow: for example, at time of decision/action/need. CDS has not reached its full potential in driving care transformation, in part because opportunities to optimize each of the five rights has not been fully explored and cultivated [25].

3.1 Right information

Right information is defined as providing the right information to end users (e.g., clinicians, patients), presenting evidence-based data that is shaped by national clinical guidelines, performance measures, and predictive analytics. The evidence-based data should be relevant to the issue at hand and actionable, meaning the information supports driving clinical actions [19, 24]. The rapid acceleration of technology and the convergence of predictive analytics and human factors address Centers for Medicare and Medicaid Services (CMS) Stage 3: Meaningful Use [26]. The process of integrating real-time analytics into clinical workflow represents a shift towards more agile and collaborative infrastructure building, expected to be a key feature of future health information technology strategies. As interoperability and big data analytics capabilities become increasingly central to crafting the healthcare information systems of the future, the need to address issues that ease the flow of health information and communication become even more important.

Without tools that select, aggregate, and visualize relevant information among the vast display of information competing for visual processing, clinicians must rely on cues by "hunting and gathering" in the EHR. Alerts that embody "right information" should provide just enough data that drives end user action, but not so much data so as to cause alert fatigue [27]. Providing too much information to the end user can spur cognitive overload, with the CDS being ignored or overridden.

In a random sample survey of 300 ambulatory care clinicians using an electronic prescribing system, attitudes towards a drug-drug interaction (DDI) alerting system were measured. In relation to the first of the five CDS rights, relevant and right information, 58% of survey respondents noted dissatisfaction with alerts being triggered by discontinued medications [28]. This dissatisfaction towards alerts that lack usefulness in the clinical environment has been noted by physicians as a potential reason for low rates of alert acceptance [29].

Recent literature has attempted to identify usability design principles relevant to CDS alerting, specifically in the context of medication alerting. Principles that directly relate to right information (first of the Five Rights) include: display relevant data within medication alerts that support the decision-making process, make actionable suggestions based on evidence but do not actively enforce those actions, and provide evidence to support the alerting system (e.g., clinical evidence, patient context, imaging) [30]. The majority of CDS systems assume the diagnostic process is completed accurately and do not provide features beyond general alerts, reminders, summary dashboards, and automated information retrieval. These solutions are not, in fact, decision support. DDI alerts are frequently used CDS alerts that are created to guide appropriate medication management in patients. DDI alerts are highly disregarded by physicians with 49–96% of safety alerts overridden [31] by the physician, which could possibly be due to alert fatigue. Alert fatigue occurs due to a variety of reasons, with patient specificity playing a role. DDI alerts that do not incorporate patient specific context hold varying levels of significance. "An interaction of little relevance to one patient may be of great relevance to another." In an ideal alert, specific patient context would be used to tailor the specific presentation of these DDI alerts based on age, comorbidities, or medication history [32].

Future innovative approaches will enhance CDS to quantify uncertainty in diagnostic problem solving and present the clinician with additional information regarding probability and likelihood of a diagnosis in the context of diagnoses with similar presentations. Diagnostic suggestions and guidelines are integrated as CDS rules that are extracted, rendered, and then delivered through CDS systems to provide clinicians with just-in-time information, for single disease states, assuming the diagnostic process is completed accurately. When the diagnosis is not immediately obvious, clinicians can use differential diagnosis support tools as an aid to rapidly identify diagnostic possibilities, but this method is highly subject to provider bias and requires manual input. More powerful and accurate analytic layers embedded into EHRs might mitigate both the cause and likelihood of errors (e.g., misdiagnosis) and could allow for more rapid, accurate diagnosis. Analytics-driven CDS can highlight areas prone to poor clinical decision making, increase our knowledge about conditions that are vulnerable to being missed and help prioritize diagnostic errors. The ultimate goal is to integrate clinical research, design, and systems engineering to develop optimized CDS systems – satisfying the information needs of clinicians as they formulate, debate, and discuss next steps in the diagnosis and clinical management of patients.

3.2 Right person

To the right person (second of the Five Rights) involves providing CDS interventions to the appropriate parties that have the capabilities to take appropriate action. Possibilities of "the right person" include: care team members, clinicians & care providers, patients & patient caretakers [16, 17].

Usability design principles related to the right person include displaying alerts to primary clinicians, as well as clinicians who do not have primary responsibility to serve as a second check. This is done by indicating to all professionals involved in the patient's care that there is information available, as well as informing the relevant care team as to how previous alerts were handled, if documented. Additional strategies include system-level alerts like the Rothman Index "quilt view" for alerting [33]. The Rothman Index is a comprehensive rating of overall patient condition in the hospital setting. The index is used at many medical centers and calculated based on vital signs, laboratory values, and nursing assessments in the EHR. In addition to patient-specific CDS, the "quilt view" assigns a risk color to each patient, providing an overall indicator of a unit's condition, available for viewing by both clinicians with primary responsibility of the patient and unit leadership (e.g., a unit's charge nurse).

Providing correct information is not limited to only clinicians but can be extended to the patient. Patient decision support interventions are attempts to use CDS to translate medical knowledge to patients. Patient facing CDS assist patients in gaining a better understanding and comprehension of medical decisions. Patient facing CDS shows great promise in assisting shared decision making between physician and provider, but there are still obstacles to overcome regarding implementation. A recent systematic review of literature related to implementation of patient decision support interventions have shown that there are administrative and clinical challenges in implementation of these patients facing CDS [34].

There is a significant push toward providing the important and informative information to the appropriate users in the clinical settings in a consistent and usable manner. The Agency for Healthcare Research and Quality (AHRQ) funded demonstration projects that yielded important knowledge about translating narrative guidelines into formats that can be used by EHRs, and about implementing CDS in clinical settings [35]. AHRQ also acknowledge a range of important research questions still to be answered in the areas of guideline translation, local CDS implementation, clinician and patient factors that affect success, and policy and sustainability issues. Rather than replicate the technical advances that have been made in the field, future research will focus on translating a CDS tool into a framework oriented towards streamlining creation, implementation, and dissemination. Most of the "work" performed by everyday clinicians for patients is highly individualized. Thus, a deep understanding of the local, highly personal context is required to get CDS "right." Moreover, getting CDS "wrong" will not be the equivalent of not providing any CDS. Rather, there is a real risk of inefficiency (e.g., interruption and distraction, leading the clinician to forget what they were thinking about before the CDS) and patient harm (e.g., acceptance of CDS that is inappropriate given the specific patient's clinical situation).

3.3 Right format

Alert and warning complexity are especially prevalent in health information technology. Despite this issue, there is little consensus on how alerts should be generated and displayed to the user [36] as well as what level of interaction is appropriate. CDS may be implemented in various formats (e.g. alerts, order sets, protocols, patient monitoring systems, info buttons). Consequently, it becomes important for implementers to identify the issues and problems they are trying to solve and choose the best format to resolve the problem at hand (third of the Five Rights). Furthermore, when developing a CDS program, implementers should create an inventory of current systems to determine which CDS tools are available, which tools need to be developed in-house, and which tools need to be purchased through a vendor. Specifically, there is a lack of knowledge regarding the most effective ways to differentiate alerts, highlighting important pieces of information without adding noise, to create a universal standard [37]. While underlying models and algorithms of CDS have been intensively studied, there remains a lack of evidence-based guidelines in terms of functional and design requirements of the system.

The purpose of an alert is to prompt an operator action. Poor alert system design has been a contributing cause of adverse events in numerous healthcare systems worldwide. The appeal of access to a large amount of clinical data must be balanced against the real possibility of information overload. Research demonstrates that medical displays are often incompatible with practitioners' workflow and unnecessarily fragment patient information [38]. Information is often spread across multiple tabs and locations that require piecemeal information search and acquisition. This may confound practitioners' ability to detect evolving changes, make it more difficult to attain a holistic view of a patient's health state, lead to care inefficiencies, and frustrate clinicians. Recognizing limits on human working memory, clinicians need external automated information systems to support early detection of patient deterioration and improve timeliness of therapeutic response. The design of alerts must improve the process of information display, reducing cognitive load on the working memory of the provider and improving the usual process that is often characterized by fragmented, non-directed information gathering.

In the absence of evidence-based guidelines specific to EHR alerting, effective alert design can be informed by several guidelines for design, implementation, and reengineering that help providers take the correct action at the correct time in response to recognition of the patient's condition [39]. In a narrative review to inform EHR alert optimization and clinical practice workflow, 42 unique recommendations were included and classified as interface, information, and interaction features [39]. The recommendations identified are described to help optimize design, organization, management, presentation, and utilization of information through presentation, content, and function. Alarm systems should be designed for and driven by human factors rather than technical capabilities. Easterby suggests seven psychological processes to be considered in display design that determine the limits of display formats: [1] detection – determining the presence of an alarm; [2] discrimination – defining the differences between one alarm and another; [3] identification – attributing a name of meaning to an alarm; [4] classification – group the alarms with a similar purpose of function; [5] recognition – knowing what an alarm purports to mean; [6] scaling – assigning values to alarms; [7] ordering and sequencing – determining the relative order and priority of alarms [40].

3.4 Right channel

Not only must a CDS provide information to the correct information to the appropriate audience in a usable format, the CDS must provide the information via the most effective and efficient channel (fourth of the Five Rights). CDS interventions can be delivered through an EHR, PHR, computerized physician order entry, an app running on a smartphone, and—if necessary—in paper form via flow-sheets, forms, and labels. Typically, organizations deploying CDS will focus very heavily on interruptive alerts—especially to physicians via computerized physician order entry (CPOE). Although alerts can be a powerful CDS intervention, they tend to be used excessively and inappropriately, resulting in commonly reported CDS problems such as alert overrides, physician frustration, and backlash. If the physician is the right person, then the EHR may be the best platform for delivering the alert. However, if a significant other is the right person, then the right platform may be a text messaging app running on a smartphone.

Emerging trends include the use of mobile technology and patient portals as CDS channels. Healthcare systems are gradually moving toward new models of care based on integrated care processes shared by various care givers and on an empowered role of the patient. Good communication between patients, their providers and caregivers improve patient satisfaction and are central to optimal outcomes. The explosion of mobile technologies and healthcare applications represents a growing opportunity to optimize care delivery. Availability of medical information through internet-enabled smartphones and tablets has increased significantly. These applications provide medical providers with recommendations for treatment, disposition, and prescriptions conforming to the most up-to-date evidence-based guidelines; allow instant access to journals and information sources at the click of a button; and deliver a plethora of CDS tools. Patients are also using the technology to communicate with their providers, research medical conditions, and become more active participants in their care. Mobile applications illustrating complex medical conditions and processes and online resources are being recommended by physicians to aid the patient in this role.

3.5 Right workflow

The clinical space is polluted with alerts that are unheeded. Despite the theoretical promise of CDS systems, their development and successful implementation is poorly managed [41]. Right workflow (fifth of Five Rights) is defined as making sure information is presented at the right time and is available when needed. For example, passive alerts can appear in a prominent place in the EHR – a decision based on the results of a workflow analysis – and can be processed once the physician completes the physical examination. An alternative method would be when the physician closes the patient record they are given a prompt informing them there are outstanding patient alerts that need to be processed. The application of human factors in determining the right workflow includes but is not limited to ethnographic research include workflow analysis and usability testing.

Workflow analysis is a process in which researchers examine the progression of workflows to improve efficiency. Ethnographic research is a qualitative method where researchers observe and/or interact with system users in their real-life environment. Observation is a systematic data collection approach by which information is gathered by watching behavior, events, and people in natural settings and naturally occurring situations. User observation is unique in that it combines the researcher's participation in the lives of the people and processes under study while also maintaining a professional distance [42]. According to Angrosino, "Observation is the act of perceiving the activities and interrelationships of people in the field setting" [43]. The demand for usability testing is becoming increasingly important as healthcare moves toward a commitment to the Triple Aim: improving the experience of care, improving the health of populations, and reducing per capita costs of healthcare. Usability testing is a critical step in informing and helping define the standard of care for healthcare system, promoting safe, high-quality care for patients. It provides the opportunity to assess user behavior, interaction, and performance data to measure how the design of medical devices, equipment, practices, and protocols affect performance, quality, workflow (cognitive and clinical), and patient safety [44, 45]. The goal is to provide evidence to support the selection and implementation of safe and user-friendly CDS, inform decision-making, and develop better solutions that update, unify, and generally improve the usability of healthcare providers' tools and systems related to optimal diagnosis and clinical management.

4. Scratching the surface of better CDS

Recent literature supports that using the Five Rights of CDS framework as a foundation for CDS design, development, and implementation can have positive impacts on CDS acceptance as well as positive outward reaching effects on clinician workflow, improved patient care, and increased patient safety.

To provide a useful, standardized, and evidence-based diagnostic aid, Kharbanda et al. developed a CDS tool to aid in the evaluation and management of treatment care for pediatric patients with suspected appendicitis in the emergency department (ED). The CDS took a three-component approach, combining: a standardized abdominal pain medication order set; a web-based stratification tool used to classify the pediatric patient as low, medium, or low-risk for appendicitis; and a "time of ordering" alert with steps for treatment and imaging guidance (e.g., medication and imaging options) for the identified level of risk [46]. The implementation of an evidenced based CDS reduced the number of costly computed tomography (CT) imaging, potentially reducing the number of unnecessary radiation exposure to developing children.

Using a Bluetooth enabled blood glucose (BG) meter in conjunction with a cloud-based clinical decision support system (CDSS), clinicians were able to increase efficiency and efficacy of glucose monitoring in diabetic patients [47]. The appropriate technology enabled patients to increase self-monitoring. Clinicians were able to more closely monitor patient's BG readings and suggest insulin dose and titration changes between appointments, as applicable, using the patient's BG meter, text message, or phone call. Use of the CDSS aided the patient's care team to increase efficiency in their workflow and provide improved patient care regarding getting patients within target glucose ranges.

In addressing the deficiencies of appropriate medication ordered for patients with impaired renal function and the lack of re-assessment of medication appropriateness as patients' symptoms change, Awdishu et al. developed a dynamic CDS tool within an EHR that provides renal medication dosing suggestions and alternative therapies suggestions at the initial time of medication prescription ("prospective alert") and temporal alerts during continuous monitoring of patients' renal function ("look-back alerts") [48]. All alerts only fired during the order entry workflow (i.e., at the point of placing and/or updating a medication order). Study results indicate the alerts had a significant impact on the selection of appropriate drug prescription during medication initiation, in addition to significant improvements for appropriate medication adjustments.

Exploring additional channels for CDS, Burgess et al. evaluated the impact of an online care processing models (CPM), on the quality of care for patients with lower extremity cellulitis (LEC). When the CPM was utilized, there was an increasing trend in appropriate drug prescription during medication initiation and at patient discharge [49].

Despite continued growth and successful implementation of CDS tools, CDS has not reached its full potential in driving health care transformation [25].

Opportunities to optimize each of the five rights continue to be highlighted by challenges and barriers such as gaining full acceptance from users from various disciplines, cultures, and use settings; continually maturing technology standards that restrict cohesive integration; and the growing resource requirements needed to keep customized solutions up to date [50].

5. Conclusions

Human factors approach underpins patient safety and quality improvement science, offering an integrated, evidence-based, coherent approach to improving the science behind health care delivery. Improvements in display management have commenced, but there is great need for further progress. As demands on healthcare providers increase (the result of increasing availability and complexity of medical devices and delivery processes, higher patient illness acuity, higher costs for process interruptions), the potential for problems are increasing. Safety-critical interactions with the EHR are especially common, challenging, and important. In safety critical environments (such as hospitals), the importance of well-designed, usable interfaces is increased precisely because of the potential for catastrophic outcomes. Time pressure, competing demands, and ambiguous alert design reduce a user's opportunity to detect signals in the face of noise and may lead to inadvertent confirmation bias. The importance of and need for appropriate user interface design is increasingly evident in such environments.

The efficiency of alert design depends on several guidelines for design, implementation, and reengineering that help providers to take the correct action at the correct time in response to recognition of the patient's condition. Hollifield proposed the following six guidelines for alert development: [1] alarms are properly chosen and implemented; [2] alerts are relevant, clear, and easy to understand; [3] operators can rapidly assess the relative importance of alerts; [4] operators can process alert information during high frequency events; [5] priority determination; and [6] alert management enhances the operator's ability to make a judgment based on experience and skill [51]. Stanton and Stammer place importance on alert prioritization and organization, which impact early detection of critical alerts [52]. Information must be presented so it is compatible with human capabilities and limitations, so that the system remains usable for the provider in all situations [21]. We considered aspects of display design in relation to taxonomy of provider psychological process that illustrate the different nature of the two types of enhanced visual display models developed for this research.

CDS can be utilized across a variety of conditions and circumstances to promote optimal care. CDS has ultimately improved adherence to recommended care standards and may result in lasting improvements in the clinical setting [53, 54]. However, the accuracy and acceptance of CDS can be limited by numerous factors, including poor usability and too many false positive alerts. There is growing evidence that health information technology interventions ultimately improve patient outcomes through early diagnosis and recommendations of evidence-based protocols [55]. The world of cognitive support is promising due the innovation and growth in this area of study.

Conflict of interest

The authors declare no conflict of interest.

Author details

Robin Littlejohn, Ronald Romero Barrientos, Christian Boxley and Kristen Miller*
MedStar Health National Center for Human Factors in Healthcare,
Washington, DC, USA

*Address all correspondence to: kristen.e.miller@medstar.net

IntechOpen

© 2020 The Author(s). Licensee IntechOpen. This chapter is distributed under the terms of the Creative Commons Attribution License (http://creativecommons.org/licenses/by/3.0), which permits unrestricted use, distribution, and reproduction in any medium, provided the original work is properly cited.

References

[1] Larosa JA, Ahmad N, Feinberg M, Shah M, Dibrienza R, Studer S. The use of an early alert system to improve compliance with sepsis bundles and to assess impact on mortality. Critical Care Research and Practice. 2012;**2012**:980369

[2] Bailey TC, Chen Y, Mao Y, Lu C, Hackmann G, Micek ST, et al. A trial of a real-time alert for clinical deterioration in patients hospitalized on general medical wards. Journal of Hospital Medicine. 2013;**8**(5):236-242

[3] Garg AX, Adhikari NKJ, McDonald H, Rosas-Arellano MP, Devereaux PJ, Beyene J, et al. Effects of computerized clinical decision support systems on practitioner performance and patient outcomes: A systematic review. Journal of the American Medical Association. 2005;**293**:1223-1238

[4] Ammenwerth E, Schnell-Inderst P, Machan C, Siebert U. The effect of electronic prescribing on medication errors and adverse drug events: A systematic review. Journal of the American Medical Informatics Association. 2008;**15**(5):585-600

[5] Wolfstadt JI, Gurwitz JH, Field TS, Lee M, Kalkar S, Wu W, et al. The effect of computerized physician order entry with clinical decision support on the rates of adverse drug events: A systematic review. Journal of General Internal Medicine. 2008;**23**(4):451-458

[6] Kawamoto K, Houlihan CA, Balas EA, Lobach DF. Information in practice systematic review of trials to identify features critical to success. BMJ. 31 March 2005;**330**(7494):765

[7] Field TS, Rochon P, Lee M, Gavendo L, Baril JL, Gurwitz JH. Computerized clinical decision support during medication ordering for long-term care residents with renal insufficiency. Journal of the American Medical Informatics Association. 2009;**16**(4):480-485

[8] Fischer MA, Vogeli C, Stedman M, Ferris T, Brookhart MA, Weissman JS. Effect of electronic prescribing with formulary decision support on medication use and cost. Archives of Internal Medicine. 2008;**168**(22):2433-2439

[9] Murphy EV. Clinical decision support: Effectiveness in improving quality processes and clinical outcomes and factors that may influence success. The Yale Journal of Biology and Medicine. 2014;**87**:187-197

[10] Eslami S, Abu-Hanna A, de Keizer NF. Evaluation of outpatient computerized physician medication order entry systems: A systematic review. Journal of the American Medical Informatics Association. 2007;**14**(4):400-406

[11] Hussey PS, Timbie JW, Burgette LF, Wenger NS, Nyweide DJ, Kahn KL. Appropriateness of advanced diagnostic imaging ordering before and after implementation of clinical decision support systems. JAMA. 2015;**313**(21):2181-2182

[12] Acquadro C, Berzon R, Dubois D, Leidy NK, Marquis P, Revicki D, et al. Incorporating the patient's perspective into drug development and communication: An ad hoc task force report of the patient-reported outcomes (PRO) Harmonization Group meeting at the food and drug administration, February 16, 2001. Value Health. September-October 2003;**6**(5):522-531

[13] Strom BL, Schinnar R, Aberra F, Bilker W, Hennessy S, Leonard CE, et al. Unintended effects of a computerized physician order entry nearly hard-stop alert to prevent a drug interaction:

A randomized controlled trial. Archives of Internal Medicine. 2010;**170**(17):1578-1583

[14] Hysong SJ, Spitzmuller C, Espadas D, Sittig DF, Singh H. Electronic alerts and clinician turnover: The influence of user acceptance. The American Journal of Managed Care. 2014;**20**(11):SP520-SP530

[15] Sittig DF, Krall MA, Dykstra RH, Russell A, Chin HL. A survey of factors affecting clinician acceptance of clinical decision support. BMC Medical Informatics and Decision Making. 2006;**1**:6

[16] Halbesleben JRB, Rathert C. Linking physician burnout and patient outcomes: Exploring the dyadic relationship between physicians and patients. Health Care Management Review. 2008;**33**(1):29-39

[17] Ratwani RM, Benda NC, Zachary Hettinger A, Fairbanks RJ. Electronic health record vendor adherence to usability certification requirements and testing standards. JAMA : The Journal of the American Medical Association. 2015;**314**:1070-1071

[18] Berner ES. Clinical decision support systems: State of the art. AHRQ Publication 90069. 2009. pp. 1-26

[19] Osheroff J, Teich JM, Levick D, Saldana L, Velasco F, Sittig DF, et al. Improving Outcomes with Clinical Decision Support: An Implementer's Guide. 2nd ed. Chicago: CRC Press; 2012. p. 323

[20] Carayon P, Wood KE. Patient safety - the role of human factors and systems engineering. Studies in Health Technology and Informatics. 2010;**153**:23-46

[21] Noyes J. Engineering Equipment and Materials Users' Association. Alarm Systems: A Guide to Design, Management and Procurement. Computing and Control Engineering. 2000;**11**(2):52

[22] The Computer-Based Patient Record [Internet]. Washington, D.C.: National Academies Press. 1997. Available from: http://www.nap.edu/catalog/5306

[23] Pritchett AR, Vándor B, Edwards K. Testing and implementing cockpit alerting systems. Reliability Engineering and System Safety. 2002;**75**(2):193-206

[24] Campbell JR. The five rights of clinical decision support: CDS tools helpful for meeting meaningful use. Journal of AHIMA. 2013;**84**(10):42-47

[25] Sittig DF, Wright A, Osheroff JA, Middleton B, Teich JM, Ash JS, et al. Grand challenges in clinical decision support. Journal of Biomedical Informatics. 2008;**41**(2):387-392

[26] McNeill D, Davenport TH. Analytics in Healthcare and the Life Sciences: Strategies, Implementation Methods, and Best Practices. Upper Saddle River: Pearson; 2014

[27] Woods DD. The alarm problem and directed attention in dynamic fault management. Ergonomics. 1995;**38**(11):2371-2393

[28] Weingart SN, Simchowitz B, Shiman L, Brouillard D, Cyrulik A, Davis RB, et al. Clinicians' assessments of electronic medication safety alerts in ambulatory care. Archives of Internal Medicine. 2009;**169**(17):1627-1632

[29] Isaac T, Weissman JS, Davis RB, Massagli M, Cyrulik A, Sands DZ, et al. Overrides of medication alerts in ambulatory care. Archives of Internal Medicine. 2009;**169**(3):305-311

[30] Marcilly R, Ammenwerth E, Roehrer E, Niès J, Beuscart-Zéphir MC. Evidence-based usability design

principles for medication alerting systems. BMC Medical Informatics and Decision Making. 2018;**18**(1):69

[31] Van Der Sijs H, Aarts J, Vulto A, Berg M. Overriding of drug safety alerts in computerized physician order entry. Journal of the American Medical Informatics Association. 2006;**13**(2):138-147

[32] Duke JD, Bolchini D. A successful model and visual design for creating context-aware drug-drug interaction alerts. AMIA Annual Symposium Proceedings. 2011;**2011**:339-348

[33] Rothman SI, Rothman MJ, Solinger AB. Placing clinical variables on a common linear scale of empirically based risk as a step towards construction of a general patient acuity score from the electronic health record: A modelling study. BMJ Open. 2013;**3**(5):e:002367

[34] Elwyn G, Scholl I, Tietbohl C, Mann M, Edwards AG, Clay C, et al. "Many miles to go.": A systematic review of the implementation of patient decision support interventions into routine clinical practice. BMC Medical Informatics and Decision Making. 2013;**13**(S2):S14

[35] Mardon R, Mercincavage L, Johnson M Jr, Finley S, Pan E, Arora D. Findings and Lessons From AHRQ's Clinical Decision Support Demonstration Projects. (Prepared by Westat under Contract No. HHSA 290-2009-00023I). Rockville, MD; 2014. Report No.: AHRQ Publication No. 14-0047-EF

[36] Phansalkar S, Edworthy J, Hellier E, Seger DL, Schedlbauer A, Avery AJ, et al. A review of human factors principles for the design and implementation of medication safety alerts in clinical information systems. Journal of the American Medical Informatics Association. 2019;**17**(5):493-501

[37] Miller RA, Waitman LR, Chen S, Rosenbloom ST. The anatomy of decision support during inpatient care provider order entry (CPOE): Empirical observations from a decade of CPOE experience at Vanderbilt. Journal of Biomedical Informatics. 2005;**38**:469-485

[38] Kong N, Heer J, Agrawala M. Perceptual guidelines for creating rectangular treemaps. IEEE Transactions on Visualization and Computer Graphics. 2010;**16**(6):990-998

[39] Miller K, Mosby D, Capan M, Kowalski R, Ratwani R, Noaiseh Y, et al. Interface, information, interaction: A narrative review of design and functional requirements for clinical decision support. Journal of the American Medical Informatics Association. 2018;**25**(5):585-592

[40] Easterby R. Tasks, processes and display design. In: Easterby R, Zwaga H, editors. Information Design. Wiley Chichester, UK: Chichester; 1984. pp. 19-36

[41] Gagliardi AR, Alhabib S, Members of Guidelines International Network Implementation Working Group. Trends in guideline implementation: A scoping systematic review. Implementation Science. 2015;**10**:54

[42] Fetterman DM. Ethnography: Step by Step. SAGE; 1998. p. 165

[43] Angrosino MV. Doing Ethnographic and Observational Research. Los Angeles, [Calif.]; London: SAGE; 2007. Available from: https://search.ebscohost.com/login.aspx?direct=true&db=cat00012a&AN=bourne.910143&site=eds-live&scope=site

[44] Mohammed S, Fiaidhi J. Ubiquitous Health and Medical Informatics: The Ubiquity 2.0 Trend and Beyond.

Hershey, Medical Information Science Reference; 2010

[45] Bien N, Rajpurkar P, Ball RL, Irvin J, Park A, Jones E, et al. Deep-learning-assisted diagnosis for knee magnetic resonance imaging: Development and retrospective validation of MRNet. PLoS Medicine. 2018;**15**(11):e1002699

[46] Kharbanda AB, Madhok M, Krause E, Vazquez-Benitez G, Kharbanda EO, Mize W, et al. Implementation of electronic clinical decision support for pediatric appendicitis. Pediatrics. 2016;**137**(5)

[47] Bode B, Clarke JG, Johnson J. Use of Decision Support Software to Titrate Multiple Daily Injections Yielded Sustained A1c Reductions After 1 Year [Internet]. 2019. Available from: https://www.glytecsystems.com/Evidence/use-of-decision-support-software-to-titrate-multiple-daily-injections-yielded-sustained-a1c-reductions-after-1-year-jdst.html

[48] Awdishu L, Coates CR, Lyddane A, Tran K, Daniels CE, Lee J, et al. The impact of real-time alerting on appropriate prescribing in kidney disease: A cluster randomized controlled trial. Journal of the American Medical Informatics Association. 2016;**23**(3):609-616

[49] Burgess MJ, Enzler MJ, Kashiwagi DT, Selby AJ, Sohail MR, Daniels PR, et al. Clinical study of an online tool for standardizing hospital care. Journal for Healthcare Quality. 2016;**38**(6):359-369

[50] Das M, Eichner J. Challenges and Barriers to Clinical Decision Support (CDS) Design and Implementation Experienced in the Agency for Healthcare Research and Quality CDS Demonstrations (Prepared for the AHRQ National Resource Center for Health Information Technology under C. Rockville), MD; 2010. Report No.: AHRQ Publication No. 10-0064-EF

[51] Hollifield B, Habibi E. Alarm Management: A Comprehensive Guide, Second Edition [Internet]. International Society of Automation; Second edition. 2010. Available from: http://www.amazon.com/Alarm-Management-Comprehensive-Second-Edition/dp/193600755X

[52] Stanton NA, Stammers RB. Alarm initiated activities: Matching formats to tasks. International Journal of Cognitive Ergonomics. 1998;**2**(4):331-348

[53] Shiffman RN, Liaw Y, Brandt CA, Corb GJ. Computer-based guideline implementation systems. Journal of the American Medical Informatics Association. 1999;**6**(2):104-114

[54] Oxman AD, Thomson MA, Davis DA, Haynes RB. No magic bullets: a systematic review of 102 trials of interventions to improve professional practice. CMAJ. 1995;**153, 10**:1423-1431

[55] Chaudhry B, Wang J, Wu S, Maglione M, Mojica W, Roth E, et al. Systematic review: Impact of health information technology on quality, efficiency, and costs of medical care. Annals of Internal Medicine. 2006;**144**:742-752

Chapter 6

An Intelligent Clinical Decision Support System for Assessing the Needs of a Long-Term Care Plan

Paul Kai Yuet Siu, Valerie Tang, King Lun Choy, Hoi Yan Lam and George To Sum Ho

Abstract

With the global aging population, providing effective long-term care has been promoted and emphasized for reducing the hospitalizations of the elderly and the care burden to hospitals and governments. Under the scheme of Long-term Care Project 2.0 (LTCP 2.0), initiated in Taiwan, two types of long-term care services, i.e., institutional care and home care, are provided for the elderly with chronic diseases and disabilities, according to their personality, living environment and health situation. Due to the increasing emphasis on the quality of life in recent years, the elderly expect long-term care service providers (LCSP) to provide the best quality of care (QoC). Such healthcare must be safe, effective, timely, efficiently, diversified and up-to-date. Instead of supporting basic activities in daily living, LCSPs have changed their goals to formulate elderly-centered care plans in an accurate, time-efficient and cost-effective manner. In order to ensure the quality of the care services, an intelligent clinical decision support system (ICDSS) is proposed for care managers to improve their efficiency and effectiveness in assessing the long-term care needs of the elderly. In the ICDSS, artificial intelligence (AI) techniques are adopted to distinguish and formulate personalized long-term care plans by retrieving relevant knowledge from past similar records.

Keywords: long-term care, personalized care services, clinical decision support system, artificial intelligence techniques, care plan

1. Introduction

Facing the unavoidable aging population, the demands for long-term care services are increasing and need to be addressed in modern society [1, 2]. In order to effectively provide long-term care to the elderly in the community, the Taiwan government proposed a 10-year long-term care project, namely Long-term Care Project 1.0 (LTCP 1.0), in 2007. The goal of the project was to establish a comprehensive community-based care system for (i) providing appropriate services to the elderly, (ii) improving the independence of the elderly, (iii) enhancing the quality of life, and (iv) maintaining autonomy and dignity [3]. Difference in gender, level of urbanization, culture, economy and health are also considered in this system. Eight services items are covered in LTCP 1.0: daily care services, transportation services, meal services, home and community-based rehabilitation services, respite

IntechOpen

care services, home nursing, rental of equipment and long-term care institution services [4]. Subsequently, the government launched a more extensive public framework, i.e., LTCP 2.0, in 2017 to increase the services coverage in the community [5]. **Table 1** shows the differences between LTCP 1.0 and LTCP 2.0, in which LTCP 2.0 expands the scope of services to optimize the front-end preventive care and to provide back-end connections to multi-target support services and home hospice services.

In order to provide high quality and affordable services, the ABC community care model with 3 tiers was established to clearly define the roles and responsibilities of healthcare parties involved in LTCP 2.0, as shown in **Figure 1** [6]. Tier A refers to a community integrated care service center for coordinating and allocating the resources of care services based on the care plan formulated by care managers. Moreover, Tier A also provides a localized delivery system that connects to Tier B and Tier C. Based on the assessment results from Tier A, Tier B, i.e. a multiple service center, provides corresponding diverse healthcare services for the public. Information from Tier A and Tier B is then sent to the long-term care station in Tier C for providing various care functions to the elderly. Therefore, the care managers in Tier A play an important role in LTCP 2.0 in evaluating the needs and formulating care plans [7]. However, it is complicated for care managers to perform the tasks of health assessment, reviewing historical health records and resources planning in a short time. In addition, it requires care managers with adequate knowledge and experience to handle these tasks. Due to the fact that in healthcare resources are as shortages in terms of staff and equipment, the implementation of care planning in

	LTCP 1.0	LTCP 2.0
Services targets	4	8
Services scopes	8	17
Financial resources	• Government funding • Medical development funding	• Government funding • Social welfare funding • Long-term service development funding
Innovative service	N/A	ABC community care model

Table 1.
Differences between LTCP 1.0 and LTCP 2.0.

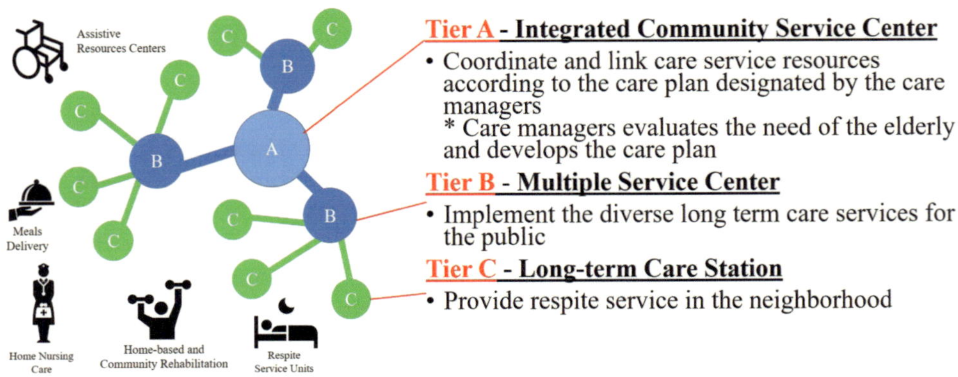

Figure 1.
ABC community care model.

LTCP 2.0 becomes challenging to achieve the goals of providing accurate and fast-responsive healthcare services.

To address the above problems, the objective of this article is to present an intelligent clinical decision support system (ICDSS) for care planning. The case-based reasoning (CBR) technique is adopted to provide the knowledge support for decision-making in care planning. By extracting the relevant knowledge from similar past cases, the care plans can be formulated in a cost-effective and time-efficient manner so as to maintain the high quality of services. The rest of article is structured as follows. Related studies and background are discussed in Section 2. Section 3 describes the architecture of the proposed system while Section 4 discusses the case study and findings. Section 5 shows the future research directions. Conclusions are drawn in Section 6.

2. Related work

Due to the development of medical technology and increased life expectancy, the number of elderly people in Taiwan is expected to increase continuously annually. According to the statistics [8], the percentage of the elderly population aged 65 or above is 13.2% in 2016. It is estimated that this population in 2026 will reach to 20.6%. Associated with the fast growth of the aging population, the reporting of chronic diseases has also increased significantly. As a consequence, the needs for long-term care services have become more demanding and urgent. In response to the increased demands for long-term care services, the government of Taiwan has considered long-term care services in healthcare industry as one of eight key industries to minimize the threats of chronic diseases [9]. Therefore, the Long-term Care Project 1.0 (LTCP 1.0) was launched in 2007 and was an initiative to integrate the home and residential-based services in Taiwan. Up to the end of 2015, over 160,000 people had received the services offered by LTCP and there are nearly 2800 institutions providing care services following the principles of LTCP. In view of the benefits offered by LTCP 1.0, a revised version of the original LTCP, i.e. LTCP 2.0, was created to further facilitate the integration of preventative care, social care and medical care in the community. In order to facilitate the implementation of LTCP 2.0 and coordinate the operation of long-term services and resources, researchers have been focusing on improving the performance of LTCP. Liu and Yao [10] adopted latent class analysis to examine the interrelationship among health indicators so as to determine the level of needs of the elderly care recipients. Lin et al. [11] studied the performance of LTCP according to the dimensions of the workforce, sources of funding, application of technology, service nature and norms. The aims of their study is to identify problems in LTCP and develop a continuous improvement strategies so as to improve the long-term care services. However, attention is rarely paid to the field of LTCP as well as providing knowledge support for decision-making. In fact, due to the shortage of knowledge manpower, it is time-consuming and tedious for care managers to effectively provide an integrated "one-stop" consultation for applications, health evaluations, care plans formulation and the coordination and delivery of long-term care services. Therefore, it is essential to provide knowledge support for decision-making processes in the care planning of LTCP.

In recent years, decision support systems have become increasingly popular for providing decision support in various industries [12, 13], and are designed to facilitate precise decision-making through the use of accurate and timely data, information and knowledge management. In the healthcare industry, the clinical decision support system is a specific term for the health customized version of decision support system [14]. The emerging clinical decision support system allows healthcare professionals to manage and manipulate the massive amount of data in an effective and efficient manner. In this situation, automatic decision-making can be provided for evaluating the health status of patients and providing corresponding treatment. Case-based reasoning (CBR) is one of the well-known artificial intelligent techniques commonly embedded in the clinical decision support system and adopts previous experience and knowledge for solving new problems [15]. The general CBR model has been formalized for computer reasoning as a four-step process: (i) retrieve the most similar case, (ii) reuse the retrieved case for solving the new problem, (iii) revise the content in the solutions if necessary, and (iv) retain the solutions as the new case stored in the case library [16]. The predictive process in the CBR allows users to takes less effort and time to generate solutions. CBR has been widely adopted in the healthcare industry in disease diagnosis, planning and resources allocations [17, 18]. Chang et al. [19] adopted CBR to develop a continuous care information system for facilitating discharge planning. By the adoption of computer-reasoning in the evaluation process of care planning, accurate continuing care solutions can be formulated in a timely manner. Wang et al. [20] developed a hybrid CBR approach to shorten the time for providing the treatment planning for the people with mental problems. Petrovic et al. [21] applied CBR in radiotherapy treatment planning to reduce the errors in planning and in recommending radiotherapy solutions. The above studies show that CBR is a promising approach in providing knowledge support for generating the solutions in the healthcare industry.

In summary, from the above literature, it is found that care managers play an essential role in the LTCP for generating appropriate and personalized long-term care solutions and in coordinating care services resources. Due to the needs for accurate and fast-responsive healthcare services, the adoption of a clinical decision support system using CBR is a feasible solution to shorten the evaluation time and improve the service quality in LTCP.

3. Methodology

In order to facilitate the decision-making of care managers, an intelligent clinical decision support system (ICDSS) is developed. The ICDSS architecture is shown in **Figure 2** and consists of three modules: (i) data collection module, (ii) case-based reasoning module, and (iii) care plan formulation module. With a systematic method to provide knowledge support for care managers, the effectiveness and efficiency in the processes of assessing the health information and formulating care plans can be improved. Consequently, accurate and fast-responsive healthcare services can be delivered to the elderly so as to maintain a high quality of care.

3.1 Data collection module

In the data collection module, the elderly with chronic diseases or disabilities can apply for the community care service through the online platform. Three types of data, historical data, medical records and personal information, are collected and uploaded to the cloud databases in electronic format. Historical data refers to past health data such as vaccination records, surgery records, and the historical data from the past public system. The medical record is the biometric data for reflecting the psychological and physiological aspects of the elderly. Heart rate, blood sugar index, vision and muscle strength are examples of the medical record. Personal information of the elderly including name, age, gender, family relationships,

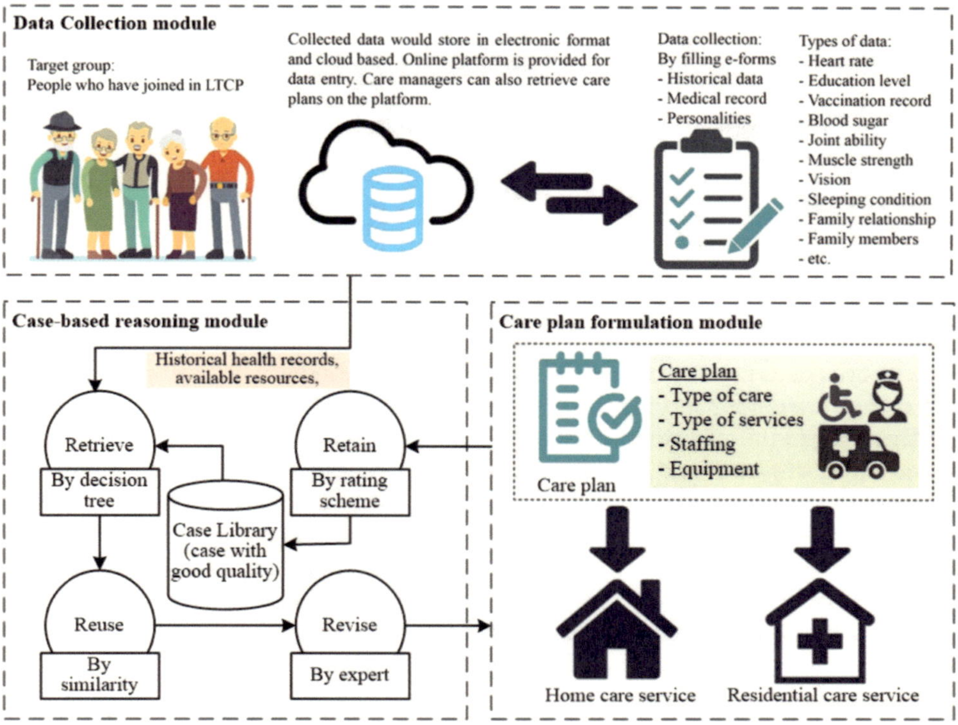

Figure 2.
An architecture of ICDSS.

personality, joint condition, sleeping ability and living environment are also collected. Apart from uploading the three types of data, an interview is conducted to understand the problems of the elderly in daily living. By doing so, care managers can collected both subjective and objective data for further data analysis in the case-based reasoning.

3.2 Case-based reasoning module

Traditionally, care managers have to review the massive amount of health data one by one for evaluating the needs of the elderly. The use of ICDSS allows care managers to effectively formulate appropriate care plans according to the needs. In this module, CBR is adopted to retrieve the most similar care records for generating the care solutions. To begin with the first stage in the CBR, i.e. case retrieval, past care records are firstly stored in the case library. An indexing tree is constructed to cluster past care records according to the key attributes that may affect the types of service provided. Along the searching path of the indexing tree, a small group of past case records are retrieved. In the reuse stage, retrieved case records are ranked descending order according to their similarity value. Eq. (1) is the expression for calculating the total similarity value.

$$\text{Total similarity value} = \frac{\sum_{i=1}^{n} w_i sim\left(f_i^I, f_i^R\right)}{\sum_{i=1}^{n} w_i} \quad (1)$$

where w_i is the weighting of the attribute i, *sim* is the function for calculating the similarity value of attributes, and, f_i^I and f_i^R are the values of attributes f_i in the new and past cases. The care record with the highest similarity value is selected and considered as the most significant reference to generate care solutions for solving the new problem. After that, care managers can make modifications to the retrieved

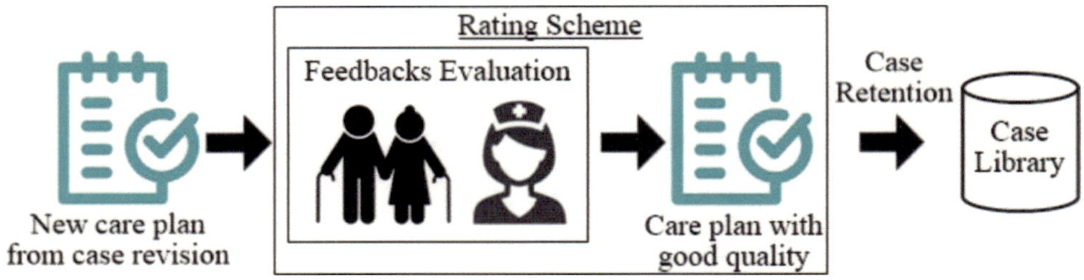

Figure 3.
Rating scheme in the case retention of CBR.

care records so as to meet the real-life situations of the elderly. Therefore, a new care plan is formulated for serving the elderly.

Differing to the traditional CBR process, a rating scheme is deployed in the case retention process to assess and monitor the effectiveness of the care plan. **Figure 3** shows the rating scheme in the case retention of CBR. As it is a long-term care service, regular meetings between care managers and the elderly or their families is required so as to collect their feedback. In addition, feedback from direct service providers, i.e. social workers and nursing staff, are also collected for the performance evaluation. Only care plans with good quality are retained in the case library for continuously improving the quality of the care records.

3.3 Care plan formulation module

After the case revision process of CBR, a new care plan with specific goals is generated. The care plan consists of several elements: (i) type of care, (ii) meals & nutrition, (iii) transportation and (iv) community center/activity recommend. According to the different nature of healthcare services, i.e. home care services or residential care services, different levels of healthcare services are provided for the elderly. In addition, details of the care plan are shared and transferred to the healthcare parties in Tier B and Tier C in the ABC community care model. Based on the care plan, operational guidelines can be provided to caregivers so as to deliver the corresponding healthcare services. Considering the health deterioration occurred in the elderly, the needs of healthcare services will move from less intensive care towards more intensive care via ABC model. Therefore, the re-evaluation of care plan is required every month to ensure its appropriateness.

4. Case example

In this section, a case example is illustrated to demonstrate the application of the ICDSS for providing knowledge support for decision-making in care planning. The case company is one of integrated community service centers located in Taichung, Taiwan. The main objective of the case company is to bring "Health and Happiness" for the elderly so as to maintain their quality of life, and physical and mental health in the community. The main staff members in the case company are care managers and supervisors such as social workers, nurses, occupational therapists and pharmacists for formulating care plan and coordinating care service resources. **Figure 4** shows the existing operation flow in the case company. The current practice of information flow, elderly health evaluation, healthcare service suggestions and follow up services are done manually. Care managers base on their experience to provide suggestions for the elderly. However, it is time-consuming and ineffective for care managers to implement these complicated steps in care planning. In

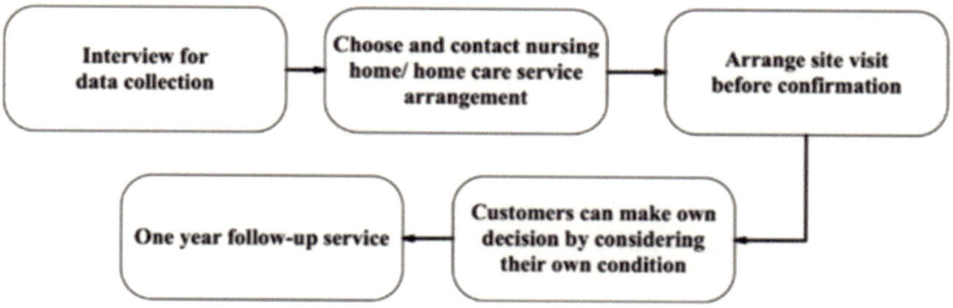

Figure 4.
Existing operation flow in the case company.

addition, human errors easily occurs in these evaluation processes, resulting in high complaint rates and poor service satisfaction in the case company.

4.1 Implementation of ICDSS

In order to tackle the above mentioned problems, the case company decided to implement the proposed system in providing knowledge support in care planning. Instead of the traditional in-person application method, the online platform is developed to collect the information. As mentioned in Section 3.1, data such as historical data, medical record and personal information are inputted by the elderly and then stored in the cloud database of the Data Collection Module. After submitting the application, care managers can note the new application in the ICDSS. An interview can be arranged to understand their current health situation and problems faced in daily living. The interview results are also stored in the database. In order to reduce the errors in the care management processes, care managers have to verify the accuracy of the data provided by the elderly.

Relevant information is then extracted and transfer to the Case-based Reasoning Module for further data analysis. In the case-based reasoning module, care managers have to identify the key attributes for constructing the indexing tree and retrieving the past care records. In this situation, five attributes: (i) kind of mobility, (ii) self-care ability, (iii) type of neuropsychiatric condition, (iv) communication method and (v) age are defined as key attributes that may significantly influence the type of services provided in care planning. **Figure 5** shows the user interface

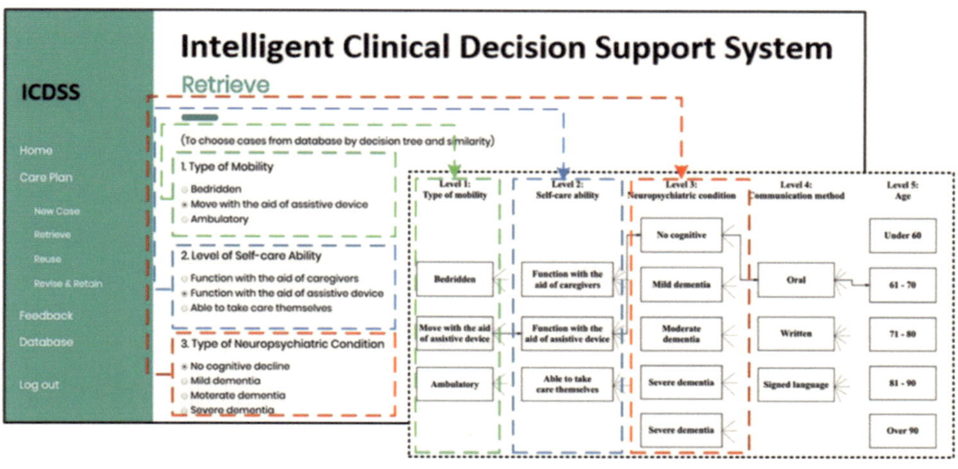

Figure 5.
The user interface for case retrieval.

for case retrieval. According to the structure of the indexing tree, the small group of past case records which match the specifications are retrieved. After that, the retrieved past case records are ranked using Eq. (1) so as to distinguish the most suitable case record. A total of 17 attributes are used to calculate the total similarity value of care records, as shown in **Table 2**. Based on the results from the case reuse, the care record with highest similarity value is extracted. An applicant is selected to illustrate the mechanism of CBR in ICDSS and details of the applicant are shown in **Table 3**. It is found that the elderly needs assistive devices for performing the movement and self-care activities. She does not have any problem of cognitive decline. A comprehensive review is implemented for deciding on the type of services. After the processes of case retrieval and reuse, the past care record (ID: 0082) has the highest similarity value (91.21%) to the new applicant. Therefore, care managers can select the past care record (ID: 0082) as the most significant reference for generating the new long-term care solutions.

To formulate a tailor-made care plan according to the needs of the elderly, modifications are made by care managers to add additional healthcare information and revise the content of the past care record. Therefore, a new care plan with services details can be generated, as shown in **Figure 6**. In the new care plan, home care services are provided to the new applicant three times per week. Therefore, this information is sent to the caregivers in Tier B and Tier C for allocating the

No.	Attributes	Weighting	No.	Attributes	Weighting
1	Living condition	1	9	Percentage of falling	2
2	Height	1	10	Drinking	2
3	Weight	1	11	Smoking	2
4	Glucose	1	12	Arthritis	2
5	Heart rate	1	13	Cancer	2
6	Upper blood pressure	1	14	Dysphagia	2
7	Lower blood pressure	1	15	Liver disease	2
8	Body temperature	1	16	Mental disease	2
			17	Urinary	2

Table 2.
Attributes for calculating the similarity value of care records.

Items	Detail	Items	Detail
Name	JL	Gender	Female
Age	69	Weight (kg)	57
Communication method	Oral	Height (cm)	160
Mobility	Move with the aid of assistive devices	Blood pressure (mmHg)	108/46
Self-care ability	Function with the aid of assistive devices	Heart rate (bpm)	80
Neuro-psychiatric	No cognitive decline	Body temperature (°C)	36.4
Living condition	Living with family	Fall (%)	18

Table 3.
Details of the applicant.

corresponding healthcare resources. In each visit, caregivers are required to measure the biometric data including blood pressure, heart rate, blood glucose level and body temperature. They have to assist the elderly in bathing and filling the drug organizer. In addition, transportation service is provided for pick from their home to the hospital for regular checking. By doing so, community-based long-term care services can be delivered.

In order to ensure the quality of care provided, a feedback survey is conducted to measure the performance of the care plan, as shown in **Figure 7**. In addition, a regular meeting is held for nursing staff participating in serving this elderly so as to discuss and understand the problems faced in delivering the healthcare services. The care plan with good quality is then retained in case library for continuously quality improvement purposes.

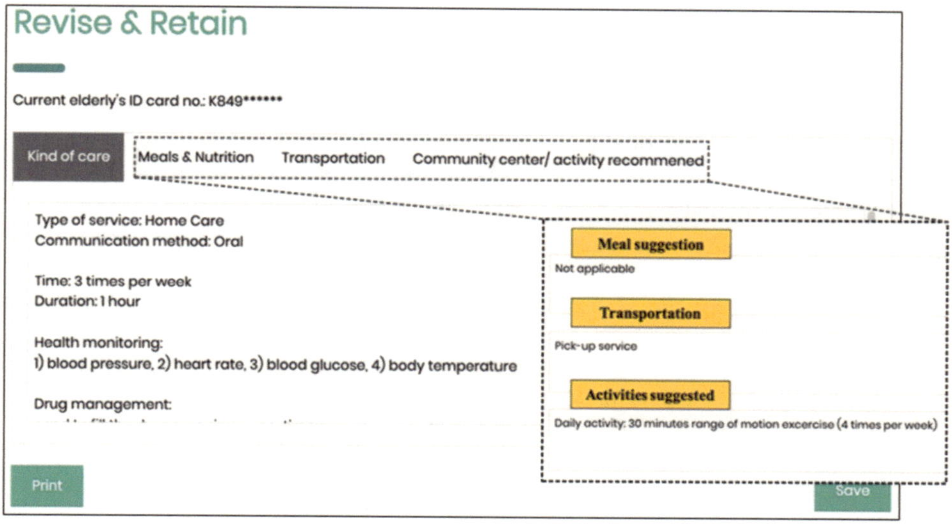

Figure 6.
The details of the retrieved past care record.

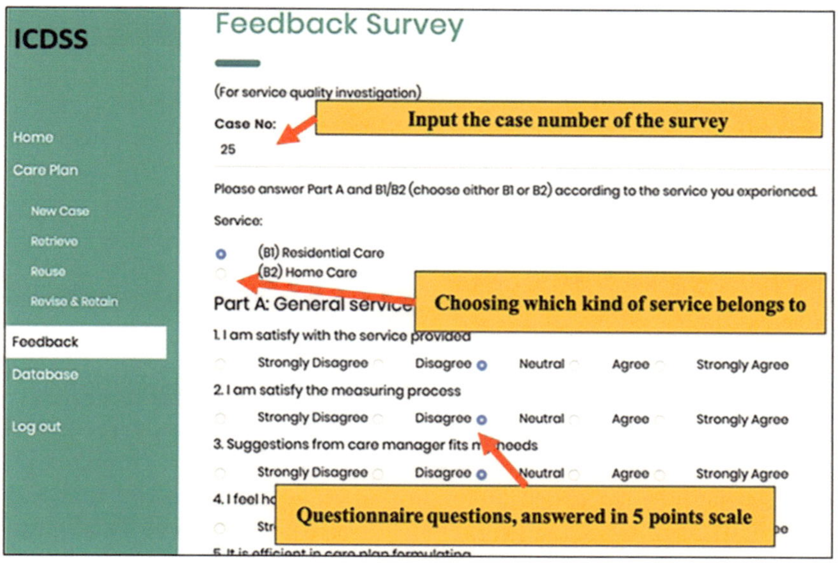

Figure 7.
Feedback survey for the elderly.

4.2 Findings

Through the pilot study in the case company, the ICDSS contributes to (i) improve the efficiency in care planning, and (ii) enhance the quality of long-term care services.

With the implementation of the ICDSS, it found that ICDSS offers several benefits to the case company. Firstly, it improves the efficiency in care planning. Instead of the traditional manual approach in care planning processes, ICDSS allows the care managers to formulate personalized long-term care solutions based on past explicit knowledge. **Table 4** shows the performance improvements after the use of ICDSS. With the use of ICDSS, care managers can review the health records provided by the elderly in the online platform rather than finding such information from separate data files. Therefore, the time for reviewing health records is significant reduced by 80.77% Moreover, the time for formulating the details of the care plan is also reduced from 156 to 22 min. Since the knowledge in past care records is extracted for solving new cases with similar problems, care managers can effectively generate solutions for providing the appropriate healthcare services and promoting the preventive health.

Furthermore, ICDSS prevents knowledge loss for formulating care plans. Since care managers with different levels of experience are employed in the case company, there may be some variations in the context of care plans. The adoption of ICDSS allows the valuable knowledge to be stored and shared in the form of past care records. Care managers, especially junior care managers, can make use of this knowledge to facilitate their decision-making. Thus, consistent long-term care solutions can be generated by different care managers. In addition, the number of complaints per week is reduced from 8 to 2. With the decrease in the number of complaints, the service satisfaction is significantly improved. Not only can the integrated community service center in Tier A enhance the service satisfaction, but also the healthcare parties in Tier B and Tier C.

Performance indicator	Without ICDSS (min)	With ICDSS (min)	Improvement (%)
Time for reviewing health records	52	10	80.77
Time for formulating the details of care plan	156	22	85.90

Table 4.
Performance improvement after the use of ICDSS.

5. Future research directions

5.1 Explore the adoption of the Internet of Things (IoT) in residential care services

According to Zhao et al. [22], there is growing evidence that chronic diseases are the major issue associated with aging population. In the last decade, the Internet of Things (IoT) is a newly emerging technology for the healthcare industry [23]. Under the IoT platform, information can be gathered, processed and analyzed to serve individual and healthcare organizations. IoT has been widely adopted in hospitals and home care services for remote monitoring and disease diagnosis. It is not only to help increase the data accuracy of the clinical decision support system, but also to provide early detection of any abnormalities occurring. In fact, its application can be further explored in residential care services. Current adoption of the IoT in nursing homes are lagging behind the hospitals and home care services providers. As one of the important long-term care service providers in LTCP 2.0, future research effort can be paid in extending the adoption of IoT in nursing homes so as to speed up its daily routine processes. Considering that numerous healthcare parties are involved in the LTCP 2.0, the IoT allows the caregivers to real-time collect and monitor the biometric data of the elderly through the equipment of the sensors. It also facilitates the information exchange among various parties. Once the abnormalities occurred, instant actions can be generated by corresponding healthcare parties to prevent the further health deterioration.

5.2 Explore a big data analytics platform for data management and manipulation

On the other hand, due to the application of smart devices and social media in healthcare services, there is an exponentially increase of health-related big data [24]. It is necessary to develop big data analytics platforms with text mining and machine learning abilities for facilitating data management and manipulation. For example, with the use of IoT, massive health data can be collected and stored in the cloud platform. The data analytic techniques such as artificial intelligence help discover the hidden pattern of available data and generate invaluable knowledge for supporting the proactive healthcare services in the LTCP 2.0. Criteria, including the ability to manipulate, continuity, ease of use, availability, quality assurance, privacy and security, should be considered in designing of this platform [25]. In addition, any data lag between data collection and processing should be avoided in this platform for achieving real-time big data analytics. Therefore, how to integrate the mentioned elements in the big data analytics platforms should be considered in future research so as to improve the effectiveness of LTCP.

6. Conclusions

To cope with the aging population, the needs for healthcare services as well as community care services are demanding. With the purpose of reducing the burden on caregivers, healthcare parties are seeking ways to better utilize the limited resources to improve the service quality. In Taiwan, LTCP 2.0 has been launched to create a comprehensive community-based care and health support system for the elderly. Care managers in Tier A play crucial roles in LTCP 2.0 for deciding on the types of service provided and in coordinating with care service resources. However, the traditional manual approach relying on care manager experience to perform the evaluation tasks and care plan formulation is ineffective. Without a knowledge-based decision support system, it is difficult for care managers, in a timely manner, to generate personalized long-term care solutions as well as coordinating care resources in Tier B and Tier C. Therefore, in this chapter, the ICDSS is designed to provide the knowledge support for decision-making in care planning of LTCP 2.0. The adoption of CBR in ICDSS approach allows care managers to disseminate the experience gained from the past similar care records. By doing so, it enables the successful execution of care planning so that fast-responsive and accurate healthcare services can be delivered. Furthermore, it enables data sharing and communication among healthcare parties in the LTCP 2.0, so that correct caring guidelines and knowledge can be transferred in a timely way to caregivers who provide direct care to the elderly timely. By so doing, the service quality can be greatly enhanced.

Acknowledgements

The authors would like to thank Research Office and Faculty of Engineering of the Hong Kong Polytechnic University through the Engineering Doctorate programme for supporting this project (Project Code: RU8J).

Author details

Paul Kai Yuet Siu[1], Valerie Tang[1], King Lun Choy[1*], Hoi Yan Lam[2] and George To Sum Ho[2]

1 Department of Industrial and Systems Engineering, The Hong Kong Polytechnic University, Hung Hom, Hong Kong

2 Department of Supply Chain and Information Management, The Hang Seng University of Hong Kong, Shatin, Hong Kong

*Address all correspondence to: kl.choy@polyu.edu.hk

IntechOpen

© 2019 The Author(s). Licensee IntechOpen. This chapter is distributed under the terms of the Creative Commons Attribution License (http://creativecommons.org/licenses/by/3.0), which permits unrestricted use, distribution, and reproduction in any medium, provided the original work is properly cited.

References

[1] He A, Chou K. Long-term care service needs and planning for the future: A study of middle-aged and older adults in Hong Kong. Ageing and Society. 2017;**1**:1-33. DOI: 10.1017/S0144686X17000824

[2] Beard HPJR, Bloom DE. Towards a comprehensive public health response to population ageing. Lancet (London, England). 2015;**385**(9968):658

[3] Executive Yuan. Long-Term Care 2.0 Plan for Greater Peace of Mind. Taipei, Taiwan: Executive Yuan; 2018

[4] Wang, H. H., & Tsay, S. F. (2012). Elderly and long-term care trends and policy in Taiwan: Challenges and opportunities for health care professionals. The Kaohsiung Journal of Medical Sciences. **28**(9):465-469

[5] Ministry of Health and Welfare. Achievements of Ten-Year Long Term Care Program. Ministry of Health and Welfare of Taiwan: Taipei, Taiwan; 2017

[6] Government of Taiwan. Earning Statistics in June 2018. In: Bureau S, editor. Statistics from Statistical Bureau. Taipei, Taiwan: 2018

[7] Yeh MJ. Long-term care system in Taiwan: The 2017 major reform and its challenges. Ageing & Society. 2019;**1**:1-18

[8] Hou SI. A Taiwan study abroad program on aging, culture, and healthcare. Educational Gerontology. 2018;**44**(1):18-27

[9] Department of Health. Taiwan Public Health Report. Taipei: Department of Health, Taiwan; 2010

[10] Liu LF, Yao HP. Examining the need assessment process by identifying the need profiles of elderly care recipients in the ten-year long-term care project (TLTCP) of Taiwan. Journal of the American Medical Directors Association. 2014;**15**(12):946-954

[11] Lin PJ, Shiue YC, Tzeng GH, Huang SL. Developing a sustainable long-term ageing health care system using the DANP-mV model: Empirical case of Taiwan. International Journal of Environmental Research and Public Health. 2019;**16**(8):1349

[12] Arnott D, Pervan G. A critical analysis of decision support systems research revisited: The rise of design science. In: Enacting Research Methods in Information Systems. Cham: Palgrave Macmillan; 2016. pp. 43-103

[13] Shibl R, Lawley M, Debuse J. Factors influencing decision support system acceptance. Decision Support Systems. 2013;**54**(2):953-961

[14] Bose R. Knowledge management-enabled health care management systems: Capabilities, infrastructure, and decision-support. Expert Systems with Applications. 2003;**24**(1):59-71

[15] Kolodner J. Case-Based Reasoning. San Mateo: Morgan Kaufmann; 1993

[16] Prentzas J, Hatzilygeroudis I. Assessment of life insurance applications: An approach integrating neuro-symbolic rule-based with case-based reasoning. Expert Systems. 2016;**33**(2):145-160

[17] Gu D, Liang C, Zhao H. A case-based reasoning system based on weighted heterogeneous value distance metric for breast cancer diagnosis. Artificial Intelligence in Medicine. 2017;**77**:31-47

[18] Marling C, Montani S, Bichindaritz I, Funk P. Synergistic case-based reasoning in medical domains. Expert Systems with Applications. 2014;**41**(2):249-259

[19] Chang CL, Cheng BW, Su JL. Using case-based reasoning to establish a continuing care information system of discharge planning. Expert Systems with Applications. 2004;**26**(4):601-613

[20] Wang WM, Cheung CF, Lee WB, Kwok SK. Knowledge-based treatment planning for adolescent early intervention of mental healthcare: A hybrid case-based reasoning approach. Expert Systems. 2007;**24**(4):232-251

[21] Petrovic S, Khussainova G, Jagannathan R. Knowledge-light adaptation approaches in case-based reasoning for radiotherapy treatment planning. Artificial Intelligence in Medicine. 2016;**68**:17-28

[22] Zhao C, Wong L, Zhu Q, Yang H. Prevalence and correlates of chronic diseases in an elderly population: A community-based survey in Haikou. PLoS One. 2018;**13**(6):e0199006

[23] Yuehong YIN, Zeng Y, Chen X, Fan Y. The internet of things in healthcare: An overview. Journal of Industrial Information Integration. 2016;**1**:3-13

[24] Raghupathi W, Raghupathi V. Big data analytics in healthcare: Promise and potential. Health Information Science and Systems. 2014;**2**(1):3

[25] Ohlhorst F. Big Data Analytics: Turning Big Data into Big Money. Vol. 65. Canada: John Wiley & Sons; 2012

Chapter 7

A Systematic Review of Knowledge Visualization Approaches Using Big Data Methodology for Clinical Decision Support

Mehrdad Roham, Anait R. Gabrielyan and Norm Archer

Abstract

This chapter reports on results from a systematic review of peer-reviewed studies related to big data knowledge visualization for clinical decision support (CDS). The aims were to identify and synthesize sources of big data in knowledge visualization, identify visualization interactivity approaches for CDS, and summarize outcomes. Searches were conducted via PubMed, Embase, Ebscohost, CINAHL, Medline, Web of Science, and IEEE Xplore in April 2019, using search terms representing concepts of: big data, knowledge visualization, and clinical decision support. A Google Scholar gray literature search was also conducted. All references were screened for eligibility. Our review returned 3252 references, with 17 studies remaining after screening. Data were extracted and coded from these studies and analyzed using a PICOS framework. The most common audience intended for the studies was healthcare providers (n = 16); the most common source of big data was electronic health records (EHRs) (n = 12), followed by microbiology/pathology laboratory data (n = 8). The most common intervention type was some form of analysis platform/tool (n = 7). We identified and classified studies by visualization type, user intent, big data platforms and tools used, big data analytics methods, and outcomes from big data knowledge visualization of CDS applications.

Keywords: systemic review, knowledge visualization, big data, clinical decision support, visual analytics, health care

1. Introduction

A clinical decision support system (CDSS) involves the use of digital information and communication technologies to bring relevant knowledge to bear on the healthcare and well-being of the patient ([1], p. 6). A CDSS has the following components ([1], p. 11):

Purpose: Task or process of clinical care which uses the CDSS.
Structure:

a. Decision Model (Organization of data and/or knowledge to generate recommendations)

b. Knowledge Base (Knowledge content used by the CDSS)

c. Information Model (Representation of clinical and decision support parameters)

d. Result Specification (Decision model output for user support)

e. Application Environment (CDSS interaction with a host application (e.g. an electronic health record system))

The growing use of medical/healthcare big data and data analytics is having a profound impact on decision models and knowledge bases in CDSS development and applications of today. There is a particular need to address user requirements when attempting to recognize patterns in the massive volumes of data being presented to decision makers (as in the Result Specification component of a CDSS structure, as outlined above). In psychology and cognitive neuroscience, pattern recognition in humans is the result of a cognitive process whereby the brain attempts to match information from a stimulus that is received and entered into short term memory with certain content retrieved from long-term memory. While the stimulus may arise from any of our senses, in this chapter we will focus on visual sensations of information that can inform decision making.

Why is knowledge visualization important to clinical decision support? Knowledge visualization is essential when there is a need to augment human capabilities rather than to attempt to automate decision-making computationally. Data mining is widely used for discovering latent knowledge from databases. This can contribute to clinical decision making. Electronic health record (EHR) and other healthcare systems contain large volumes of patient data, often with different formats and structures, so these data are typically accessible only in a form that is not conducive to rapid synthesis and interpretation for potential therapeutic outcomes.

Medical data inherently contain information that provides support for patient-centric and personalized healthcare. Machine learning approaches, combined with high-performance distributed computing technologies such as Hadoop can assist in the exploitation of big healthcare databases. In a high pressure clinical environment, well-designed knowledge-based visualization can play a key role for clinicians and managers who must deal with complex issues and decisions. These may arise from algorithms derived through computational results from healthcare databases containing data from many patients, with each record having hundreds of attributes. As other chapters in this book discuss in detail, there are machine learning/deep learning and other approaches that can convert these massive databases into decision support resources. These resources are virtually never deterministic and are difficult to validate to a high degree of accuracy, but they can help to support decision makers needing to make individualized healthcare decisions.

The value in knowledge visualization lies in presenting knowledge to the user in a way that gives the user factual information that is useful for current decisions. Since there are multiple dimensions to every specific decision, the visualization designer must provide flexibility in potential displays, while taking into account limitations on computer resources, human capabilities, and the display environment. Visualization system usage can be analyzed in terms of why the user needs it, what data is shown, and how the display idiom is designed ([2], p. 1).

The digitization of patient health records has profoundly impacted medicine and healthcare. The compilation of medical history provides a holistic account of patient condition, family history, social determinants, procedures, and medications. In addition to regular treatment benefits, the availability of this information in digital form has created opportunities for population-level monitoring and studies that can help to guide initiatives for improving quality of care. Each hospital client population base varies in geography, size, and organizational structure, and extracting meaning from the data to support a hospital's strategic mission requires a combination of clinical, statistical, and technical literacy. Effective visualization of data resources is essential to the efficient use of these resources by the healthcare facility [3].

The objectives of this study are:

- To explore the sources of big data in knowledge visualization for clinical decision support;
- To identify the visualization and interactivity approaches that have been used in the light of recent CDSS advances in the use of big data;
- To identify big data analytical techniques and technologies uses in CDSS with knowledge visualization;
- To determine the purposes of CDSS, and to illustrate the potential benefits of big data and knowledge visualization for these purposes;
- To recognize what appears to be the future of visualization in the support of big data and CDSS

By systematically investigating these objectives in detail, this systematic review will make a significant contribution towards understanding how big data knowledge visualization can be used in clinical decision support. This will benefit the development of future applications in this field.

2. Methodology

2.1 Design

This systematic review was carried out according to the recommendations and reporting specified in the Preferred Reporting Items for Systematic Reviews and Meta-Analyses (PRISMA) statement [4, 5].

2.2 Inclusion and exclusion criteria

Any peer-reviewed studies published from January 2008 to April 2019 that explored the applications of big data knowledge visualization in a clinical decision support setting were retained for full-text review. Excluded studies included reports on results of: abstracts, surveys, focus groups, feasibility studies, monitoring devices, "what-if" analysis, big data collection techniques, commentaries, letters, editorials or short reports, mere usage of big data technologies or knowledge visualization, and studies not published in English. Publications describing big data and visualization applications that were not developed for clinical decision support were also excluded.

2.3 Search strategy and screening process

We developed the search strategy according to the Cochrane Handbook of Systematic Reviews of Interventions [6]. Search keywords (terms) were grouped into three categories: big data, knowledge visualization, and clinical decision support (see **Table 1**). Searches were conducted in electronic databases: EBSCOHOST, EMBASE, MEDLINE VIA OVID, PUBMED, IEEE XPLORE, WEB of SCIENCE, and GOOGLE SCHOLAR (the latter for a gray literature search) on April 5–6, 2019. We also used the related article function in PubMed, Science Direct, and Springer Link databases on initially included studies to identify additional studies.

Studies were selected in two steps. First, the title and abstract for each study were screened for inclusion and exclusion criteria and classified by two reviewers. If the title and abstract did not provide enough information to assess its relevance or if a final decision could not be made, we assessed the full article. Second, the full texts of the studies without enough information and/or deemed to be potentially relevant were reviewed randomly by two reviewers. Any disagreements between the two reviewers were resolved via discussion or by consultation with a third reviewer. Studies cited in eligible articles were also reviewed following a similar screening process. The studies identified for systematic review were examined by two reviewers qualitatively, as described below.

2.4 Data: collection, management, analysis and classification

All reviewers used a shared spreadsheet template to classify and summarize eligible studies and keep track of review progress. Counts and percentages were based on the databases from which each study was identified in the following order: WEB OF SCIENCE, IEEE XPLORE, PUBMED, EMBASE, EBSCOHOST and GOOGLE SCHOLAR. For example, if a study was identified in both WEB OF SCIENCE and EMBASE, it counted as being found within the WEB OF SCIENCE.

All eligible studies were classified using the Population/Problem–Intervention–Comparison–Outcomes–Study (PICOS) design framework [6, 7], which provides a common approach for detailed specification of the review questions and criteria during

KEYWORDS: (P) AND (I) AND (O):	
within each group the keywords are combined using the "OR" operator	
P (BIG DATA)	BIG DATA
I (KNOWLEDGE VISUALIZATION)	KNOWLEDGE VISUALIZATION OR VISUAL ANALYTICS OR INFORMATION VISUALIZATION OR VISUALIZATION OR BUSINESS INTELLIGENCE OR BI OR DASHBOARD
O (CLINICAL DECISION SUPPORT)	CLINICAL DECISION SUPPORT OR CLINICAL DECISION MAKING OR DECISION SUPPORT SYSTEMS OR HEALTHCARE OR HEALTH CARE OR HEALTH OR CARE OR CLINICAL INTELLIGENCE OR HOSPITAL OR CLINIC OR CLINICAL OR MEDICAL OR DIAGNOSIS OR TREATMENT

Table 1.
Search terms used to identify publications related to knowledge visualization of big data for clinical decision support.

study design. In this systematic review, the same PICOS categories are used to synthesize the data extracted from eligible studies. All PICOS subcategories were identified and classified through the review process. Similarly [7] where applicable, pre-existing taxonomies such as interaction taxonomy [8, 9], major date types of big data in health care [10] and target audience [7] were integrated with the PICOS framework.

The synthesis of the findings contains results for each PICOS category (Population/Problem–Intervention–Comparison–Outcomes–Study Design) which covers all related subcategories.

3. Results

A total of 2338 references were retrieved from our first search of electronic databases. A second search of the gray literature via GOOGLE SCHOLAR (n = 780) and a third manual search (n = 134) yielded a total of 3252 studies. We then removed 866 (26.6%) duplicate studies. We screened all titles and abstracts for 2386 (73.4%) papers and excluded 1843 studies because the visualizations discussed were not for healthcare, studies were only for big data without visualization or were not for CDS (clinical decision support), papers that used genomics/DNA or image data, or presented only an abstract. The full text of each of the remaining 543 (16.7%) studies was then read. A search of citations yielded an additional 34 eligible studies. A total of 577 studies were classified and 560 of these studies were excluded. The PRISMA flow diagram (**Figure 1**) summarizes the screening process. The 17 studies remaining were included in the qualitative synthesis [11–27] that follows.

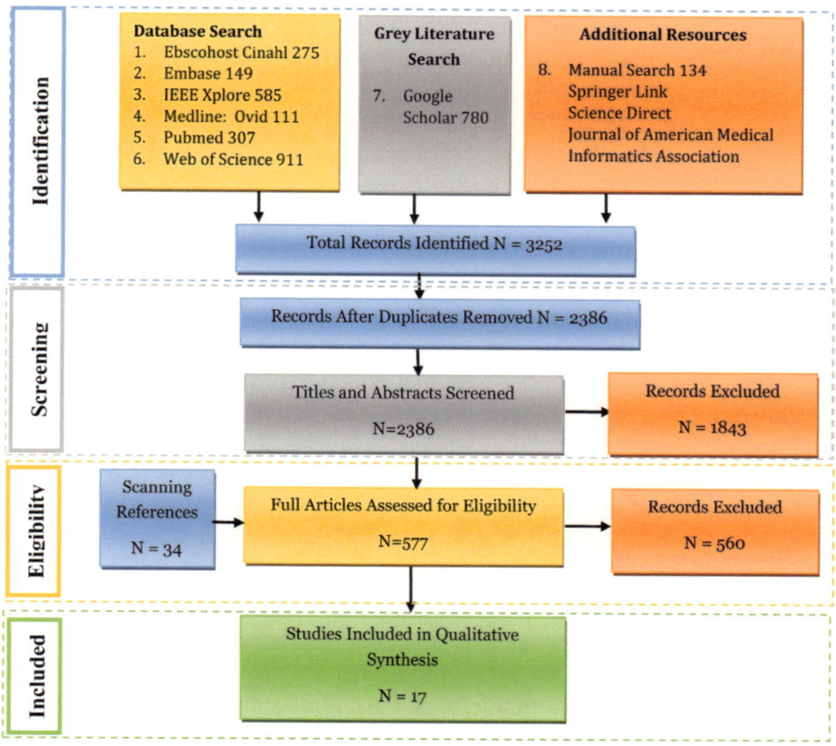

Figure 1.
PRISMA flow diagram.

3.1 Characteristics of included studies

The majority of the 17 included publications were indexed in the Web of Science (n = 12, 70.6%). The series Lecture Notes in Computer Science (LNCS) and the Journal of the American Medical Informatics Association (JAMIA) were the other sources of the studies (n = 3 (17.6%) and n = 2 (11.8%) respectively). More than half of the studies (n = 9, 52.9%) were journal publications and nearly 94% of the studies were published in the past 4.5 years (2015–2019). Studies originated from 10 countries: the USA tops the list with 9 (near 53%) publications, followed by Canada with 3 (17.6%), France and UAE with 2 each (11.8%), and Greece, Italy, South Korea, Portugal, Taiwan and Spain with 1 each (5.9%). 5 (29.4%) studies were conducted in two countries and more than half of the studies were conducted at a university. More than 82% of the studies discussed one specific type of visualization tool or system.

3.2 PICOS classification: part 1: population, patient and problem

3.2.1 Population (target users) and patients

We identified four main groups of users of big data visualization applications for clinical decision support: (1) academicians (clinical researchers and clinical epidemiologists, nurse educators) [11, 12, 17, 18, 26], (2) administrators (hospital administrators and managers) [12, 17, 25], ancillary staff (caretakers, lab managers, pharmacists) [11, 13, 25]; (3) health care providers (clinicians, nurses, physicians) [11–16, 18–27] and (4) patients [11, 14, 22, 23]. More than 94% of the studies (n = 16) were developed to support clinical healthcare provider decision-making.

A majority of the studies were in non-intensive hospital settings (n = 9, 53%), 2 in intensive surgical and trauma settings, 2 for outpatients, and 6 studies that did not specify hospital settings. Studies were designed to investigate different diseases or health problems, such as acute kidney injury [20], appendicitis [16], cardio, respiratory, and adverse events [19, 26], chronic diseases and diabetes [11, 13], hospital infections and sepsis [20, 25]. Two studies were developed to help predict various hospital complications after treatment [17, 20], and seven studies (41%) did not provide any information about specific patient diseases or problems.

3.2.2 Big data major types and sources

Big data in health care can be classified into four major types based on data sources: (1) big data in medicine, (or medical/clinical big data); (2) big data in public health and behavior; (3) big data in medical experiments; and (4) big data in medical literature [10]. We identified three major types of big data in reviewed studies (**Figure 2**).

Big data in medicine and clinics includes big data generated in hospitals, such as electronic health records (EHRs)/medical records (EMRs), personal health records (PHRs), and medical images (visual information of the internal human body). This group was the most frequent source of data in the 17 studies. Sixteen studies (94%) used big data from medicine and clinics. EHRs, EMRs (n = 12) and PHRs (n = 7) were the main sources of big data. These records consisted of some combination of clinical notes, laboratory and image reporting results, medical histories, hospital stay information, medication and allergies, patient demographics, diagnoses, sensor data, etc., all of which are the basis for personalized medicine.

Big data sourced from public health and patient activities are the second major sources of big data in our studies (n = 13, 76%). These focus on the physiological

BIG DATA TYPES	GROUP	BIG DATA AQUISION GROUP	BIG DATA AQUISION SOURCE
BIG DATA IN MEDICINE AND CLINICS	1	Electronic health record (EHR)/ electronic medical record (EMR)	Clinic or inpatient notes Clinic or inpatient notes (not for vis, only for evaluation) Clinical data from outpatient visit Clinical diagnosis Drug administration Electronic reports Hospital information resource (information about ward, bed, edc) Hospital stay Information((LOS, mortality, Length of ICU, septic shock, etc.) not for vis, only for evaluation) Identification information of patient Imaging report Information of patient Notes from physician Patient demographics (not for vis only for evaluation) Patient transfers to different hospital units (including emergency, ICU, surgical suite or ambulatory) Physical examination Physical examination (not for vis, only for evaluation) Sensor data (Glucose, Weight, Hemoglobin A1c, Medications dosage, Food/Activity Log, etc.) Sensor data (blood pressure) Surgery's work/protocols Treatment
	2	Personal health record (PHR)	Illnesses and hospitalizations Laboratory test results Laboratory test results (not for vis, only for evaluation) Medical history Medication data Medication history Medications and dosing Nursing assessments Patient demographics Provided by Government, Hospital or other organization
	3	Medical images (visual information of interior human body)	X-ray
BIG DATA IN PUBLIC HEALTH AND BEHAVIOR	4	Measures and records of the electrical and electromagnetic signals from the body	A live data feed from patients' continuous monitoring systems Continuous activity data from a wearable device (Fitbit) Continuous physiologic data from the bedside monitors Electrocardiograph (ECG) signal Electroencephalography (EEG) signal Sensor data from The Internet of Things (IOT): the approach of connecting real- world objects "to the Internet via sensors, and microprocessor chips that record and transmit data"such as brain activity, heart rate, sound waves, and body temperature Sensor data(Glucose, Weight, A1c, Medications dosage, Food/Activity Log, etc.)
	5	Vitals	Acute Physiology and Chronic Health Evaluation(APACHE) score (not for vis, only for evaluation) Temperature, pulse, respiratory rate, and blood pressure
	8	Microbiology/Pathology Laboratory	Blood glucose, carbohydrates, medications, insulin, physical activity, blood pressure, body weight,Hemoglobin A1c levels Hemoglobin A1c levels
BIG DATA IN MEDICAL LITERATURE AND SOCIAL MEDIA	12	Structured knowledge	MeSH and International Classification of Diseases 10th revision (ICD-10), etc
	13	Social Media Data	Community Forums, Social Connectivity, Meal Plans, Food and Fitness Guides,Disease Guides, Health Information

Figure 2.
Major types of big data in the 17 chosen studies.

data of users that are often collected by portable equipment [10] such as electrical and electromagnetic signals from body vitals collected by wearable devices, daily health records, and from sports and personal diets.

The main sources of the big data in public health and behavior include measures and records of electrical and electromagnetic signals from the body (n = 5, 29%) which comprise live data feeds from patient monitoring systems, electrocardiograph (ECG) and electroencephalography (EEG) signals, and sensor data from the Internet of Things (IOT). These approaches connect humans "to the Internet via sensors, and microprocessor chips that record and transmit data" such as brain activity, heart rate, sound waves, and body temperature" [22, 23].

Structured knowledge, such as big data from the medical literature under Medical Subject Headings (MESH) codes, the International Classification of Diseases 10th revision (ICD-10), laboratory test codes, etc. and social media data are also significant source of big data in a number of the 17 studies we selected for review (n = 3, 18%) (**Figure 2**).

3.2.3 Big data size

The studies reviewed included more than 5.4 million patients, mostly admitted to hospital. The sample size of patients in the studies ranged from 1757 to 2.9 million. Authors reported the number of records, tests and patient stay days that ranged from 15,700 to 17.8 million. Three studies [11, 18, 21] used structured and/or social media big data ranging from 7000 to 300 million records. About 65% of the studies (n = 11) used real time data such as ECG streaming, producing 500,000 messages per minute and 80 different types of vitals totaling 100,000 messages [26].

3.2.4 Big data types

Big data visualization studies varied significantly among the data types they could handle [8].

The data information types could be categorical (nominal (diagnosis, treatment)) or ordinal ("high", "low" blood pressure level), numerical (for example, cholesterol measure, temperature), texts, maps or networks. All 17 studies used categorical and numerical data information types, while more than 75% (n = 13) used text data types (clinician notes, laboratory results, notes, etc.). Applications in 13 studies used time series data, including real time signals in three studies (18%) [21, 22, 26]. Three studies [13, 15, 16] used maps in their applications to provide clinical decision support. All applications reviewed could deal with several types of data information, with the most common being combinations of categorical, numerical, text and time series.

We further categorized data by medical information type. Most of the studies dealt with physical examination of patients, patient outcomes and diseases, symptoms, and treatment problems which require support for clinical decision making (see **Table 3**).

A variety of data collection methods were used, with more than half of the studies using data from EHR/EMR systems. The other most common method involved receiving data from continuous monitoring via EEG, ECG, bedside monitoring, or IOT [11, 14, 19, 22, 23, 26]. Two studies used big databases [11, 20], one study used data from a provincial pathology laboratory [13] and one study used user input data in combination with IOT data [14].

3.3 PICOS classification: part 2: intervention

3.3.1 Intervention type and big data visualization techniques

We identified 11 subcategories of the PICOS intervention classification to help classify all interventions in the studies such as intervention type, big data visualization techniques, visualization types and others.

Seven studies had developed data analysis platform/tools to help the target audience (healthcare providers, academicians, etc.) [12, 16, 17, 21, 24–26]. Three studies developed and used mobile care coordination [14, 15, 20], four studies designed web portals for healthcare providers [11, 13, 22, 23] and patients [11]. Two studies used a multi-patient surveillance system [12, 18] and one study used a multi patient dashboard to support clinical decisions.

For big data visualization techniques 47% (n = 8) of all studies developed web application and 41% (n = 7) of all studies used dashboards for supporting clinical decisions.

3.3.2 Visualization types

We classified visualizations (36 different types) into 7 visualization categories (**Table 2**). On average, studies used three different visualization types. One study [21] used only one visualization type (tabular), five studies (29%) presented two different visualization types (multidimensional and tabular, tabular and temporal, etc.) [15, 17, 18, 20, 24].

PICOS subcategory: visualization types	All studies	All studies, %
3D/volumetric	3	17.6
Icons	5	29.4
Maps	3	17.6
Multidimensional	12	70.6
Tabular	14	82.4
Temporal	10	58.8
Textual	4	23.5

Visualization types subcategory.

Table 2.
PICOS classification of all publications: part 2: intervention.

In 6 studies (35.3%) three different types of visualizations were used [11, 12, 14, 25–27] with the most common combination being multidimensional, tabular and temporal. Four studies (23.5%) presented four different types of visualization [13, 16, 19, 22], but only one study used six of the seven visualization categories we identified [23].

The most common visualization category (n = 14.82%) for our studies was tabular (table) visualization for seven studies [11, 14, 16, 17, 20, 26, 27]. Three studies used tabular visualization with color (9 different indicators) and tabular visualization with color indicating risks [12, 22, 23]. One study used tabular visualization with color coding indicating change from previous state [25] or tabular visualization with color coding indicating change in value and out of normal ranges or trend of changes [21]. One study used a very innovative tabular visualization with color comets [19], where the comet head representing risks at the current time, and a tail that is 3 h long.

More than 70% of the studies (n = 12) used multi-dimensional visualization techniques such as area charts (color grading/without color grading) [14, 19, 26], bar graphs [11, 13, 14, 16, 26], bipartite graphs [25], box plots [17], bubble charts [12], causal network visualizations and heatmaps [13], key performance indicators (KPIs) [12, 16], line graphs [11, 19, 24], pie charts [11, 14, 20] and scatter plots [23].

Temporal or timeline visualization is another major category of knowledge visualization for clinical decision support (n = 10, 59%). Two studies reported visualization of just simple time series graphs without color coding [23, 24], although six studies used time series line graphs with color coding indicating: different indicators [25, 27], different status [18, 19], changes from previous encounter (Emergency, Hospital Unit, Surgery) [18] or time changes (breakfast, lunch, dinner, etc.) [11]. Four studies (24%) presented visualizations of the time series trend line [14, 16, 18, 26].

Five studies used icons [12] or icons with color grading zones [15, 19, 22, 23], three studies used 3D visualizations [13] or 3D brain maps [22, 23]. The spatial context of the big data was presented via maps [16] and interactive geo-spatial maps [13, 15]. Four studies presented textual information using simple text [18, 22, 23] or word clouds for problem identification [27]. More information about specific techniques, including background, explanations, and concepts can be found in [28].

3.3.3 Support for user intent

Information visualization can be compared and classified by interaction features. There are a great variety of interaction visualization techniques [29], but we will use an intent model proposed by [9] and extended by [8]. The concept focuses

PICOS subcategory: user intent	All studies	All studies, %
Select: mark something as interesting	15	88.2
Explore: show me something else	13	76.5
Reconfigure: show me a different arrangement	13	76.5
Encode: show me a different representation	7	41.2
Abstract/elaborate: show me more or less detail	12	70.6
Filter: show me something conditionally	14	82.4
Connect: show me related items	10	58.8
Print, submit feedback, record/download: show me something to save	8	47.1

User intent subcategory.

Table 3.
PICOS classification of all publications: part 2: intervention.

on 'What a user wants to achieve' and described as "user intent," quite effective technique to classify the low-level interaction techniques into seven descriptive high-level categories [9]. We also added an additional category that includes printing, submitting feedback or saving features (**Table 3**).

Most of the studies support user interactivity (n = 15, 89%). *Select: mark something as interesting* interaction techniques such as keeping track or managing a group are available in 15 and 13 studies respectively (77%). The *Filter*: (*show me something conditionally* interaction technique was very useful for multiple patient applications/systems and enables users to change the set of data items conditionally (in some specific conditions). This second intent played a leading part in the reviewed applications and was used in 14 studies (82%).

The *Explore: show me something else* includes items such as reposition, sorting, editing, adjusting axis and *Reconfigure: show me a different arrangement* (switch representation technique, vary visual encoding) intents were available in 13 studies (77%), while *Abstract/Elaborate: show me more or less detail* intent gives users the ability to adjust the level of abstraction of a data representation (for example via time or time constraints) is available in 12 studies (71%).

In more than half of the studies (n = 10, 59%) the *Connect: show me related items* intent is supported, where the most common interaction technique was to show patient/group relationship (n = 9, 53%). *Print, Submit Feedback, Record/Download: show me something to save* (printing, submitting feedback and recommendations, recording or downloading) intent is enabled in 8 studies (47%) with the most common being printing. *Encoding*: *show me a different representation* (temporal data binning, altering fundamental representation of visual appearance (e.g. color, size, and shape) intent is supported in 7 studies (41%) with the most common being the switch representation technique (n = 5, 29%).

3.3.4 Cognitive presentation and units visualized

In most of the 17 studies, color and similarity (grouping) are the most supported cognitive presentations. Eight studies (47%) support all cognitive presentation types, such as color, size and similarity (grouping), seven studies (41%) used color and similarity (grouping) and only one study [20] supported color and size. In just one study [15], only color presentation is supported.

More than 76% of the studies (n = 13) supported visualization for single patients, nine studies (53%) enabled visualization for multiple patients. Nearly

30% of the studies (n = 5) visualized aggregated data, such as groups of patients. Application or visualization tools can be used for single users in one study [23]. In addition, only one study supported data for multi-products [25].

3.3.5 Big data analytics methods and problems

Three main groups of analytical methods were identified in the 17 studies. The most commonly used type was Descriptive (n = 16, 94%) which summarizes data to provide useful information and sometimes prepares it for further analysis. Predictive analytics (conditional logistic regression, deep learning, machine learning, data mining, AI) was the second most popular analytical method and was used in 11 studies (65%). Only two studies (12%) supported natural language processing (text mining, sentiment analysis).

These analytical methods were used to solve a variety of analytical problems such as analyzing all note types from different providers [27], classification [23] and pattern recognition [11], clustering [13, 23], electronic risk visualization of respiratory and cardiovascular events [19], identification of sequences of inappropriate drug administration cases [21], calculation of aggregated score and progression of the patient [26], perioperative risk prediction and visualization [20], and risk estimation [17, 18, 26]. One study [24] supported only summary statistics for contours (as in box-whisker, i.e. mean, median, percentiles 25 and 75, and outliers). One other study [25] used statistical measures such as prevalence and incidence of microorganisms, antibiotics, and microbiologicals.

3.3.6 Big data platforms and tools

The use of big data requires the support of new analytical and other types of tools for handling such massive and different types of data as well as technological innovations for data management, integration and interoperability, storage, distributed processing and analysis, and visualization. The studies we reviewed used a great variety of big data platforms and tools. We classified them into 13 categories which are presented in **Table 3**.

Cloud computing services (such as Amazon Web Services, Azure and Google clouds or other clouds not specified) were used in most of the studies (n = 11, 65%).

More than half of the studies (n = 9, 53%) supported big data maintenance/storage technologies based on NoSQL databases [13] and the Hadoop Distributed File System (HDFS) [13, 20, 25, 26]. This group also included studies using Apache HBase [13, 14, 27], Cassandra [20] and MongoDB [14, 15, 17, 24].

Big data maintenance/storage technologies based on SQL and SQL on Hadoop solutions were supported in six studies. The most frequent solutions used were MySQL [17, 22], PostgreSQL, Oracle or Microsoft SQL [21, 25], RSQL [18], Spark SQL [20], Apache Hive and Apache Impala [25].

Big data scalable distributed processing and analysis was supported in 10 studies (59%) and included Hadoop MapReduce [13, 15, 22, 23, 25, 27], Apache Spark [13, 14, 20, 25, 26], Apache Mahout [23, 25], Apache Kafka [26], Elasticsearch Engine [24], Pentaho [25] and TensoronSpark [20].

We also identified studies that supported a microservices architecture for big data applications [20], big data cluster resource management [13], big data integration and interoperability and data maintenance/storage technologies (Rest for Traditional Storage (RAID)) [26], messaging cloud based services such as Google Cloud Messaging (GCM) [13] and Java Message Service (JMS) [25], mobile application development framework [22].

PICOS subcategory: comparators	All studies	All studies, %
Concurrent Controls with No Visual	1	5.9
Different Users	1	5.9
Other System/Visualization	7	41.2
Other Web Portals/Social media websites	1	5.9
None	7	41.2

Table 4.
PICOS classification of all publications: Part 3. Comparison.

Twelve studies (71%) also used non-big data analytic tools and technologies, such as i2b2 platform [21], JavaScript Object Notation (JSON) [22–26], Java Database Connectivity (JDBC) [17], Mathlab [23], NetBeans [22] and Python [20]. Six studies (35%) used R/R Server, and/or Shiny [13, 16–20] for their analyses and two studies reported using technologies to implement client-side solutions (Java, WebView, HTML, etc.) [22, 23].

3.4 PICOS classification: part 3: comparison

Table 4 presents the results of a PICOS Category Comparison. Seven studies (41%) provided or mentioned some description that compared them with another system and/or visualization tool [14, 18, 21, 23, 25–27].

Other studies provided comparison for concurrent controls with no visualization [19], different users [13], other web portals [11]. Seven studies (41%) did not provide or mention any comparison or comparators.

3.5 PICOS classification: part 4: outcomes

We identified six subcategories of the PICOS classification of outcomes (clinical decision support) which helped us to classify all outcomes in our studies such as system/tool type, clinical decision support purpose, clinical area support, measured outcome, clinical or patient outcomes divided into clinical and usability, outcomes effects or potential effects.

3.5.1 System/tool type

A majority of studies (n = 16, 94%) used decision support systems, six studies (35%) were designed for monitoring intelligent systems (sensors, devices), two (12%) used expert systems together with decision support systems [12, 25], one used a system for optimizing operations (lab resources depending on order volumes and treatments) and a decision support system [13], while only one study was developed as a visualization system [17].

3.5.2 Clinical decision support purpose

Each of the systems was designed to address a different purpose, and some were used for several purposes. We classified clinical decision support purposes into three categories of use: (1) early detection of diseases; (2) improvement of decision making; and (3) patient-centric care.

Improvement of decision making. This was the largest common purpose group (n = 14, 82%). The intent of these systems included utilizing diverse data to provide automated and augmented insight, discovery, and evidence-based health and wellness decision support (n = 10, 59%) [11, 12, 14, 16, 18, 20, 22–25], followed by monitoring and assisting individuals with intelligent systems: sensors, devices and robotics, to maintain function and independence (n = 2, 12%) [14, 15], improving accuracy [15, 24], supporting clinical workflow [27] and monitoring clinical pathways [24]. Other purposes included recalling all similar patients from an institution's electronic medical record (EMR) repository, exploring "what-if" scenarios, and collecting these evidence-based cohorts for future statistical validation and pattern mining [24]. Also included were detecting inadequate treatments [21], tracking treatments [13], supporting and formulating guidelines (standards of care, expert standards, best practices) adherence to and formulating guidelines for interpreting and adjusting severity thresholds regarding the measurement of test results [11, 13].

Early detection of diseases. This was the second most frequently used common purposes group (n = 12, 71%). The major purpose was disease monitoring, such as supervising (the patients), monitoring (the clinical condition) and notifying (healthcare personnel) [12, 17, 25, 26], reporting on continuous updates on seizures [23], visualizing signal data on physician and clinician smartphone devices to analyze, inspect, and recommend the appropriate medical decisions [22, 23], assisting users in the prescription of appropriate empiric or targeted antibiotic treatments [25]. Other purposes in this group included adopting and tracking healthier behaviors [11, 21], monitoring patient safety for adverse events following medical procedures [17], identifying VAE (ventilator adverse events) risk for more rigorously identification of adverse events at an earlier stage [26], surveillance and management of antibiotics [24], health tracking [25, 27], and surgery risk assessment [20].

Patient-centric health care was supported in two studies (12%). This included planning post-discharge care coordination (which could include the follow-up visit with the primary care physician or with a subspecialist, or care on subsequent days at home by a visiting nurse) [16] and cyber-based empowering of patients and healthy individuals to play a substantial role in their own health and treatment [11].

3.5.3 Clinical area support

We further categorized our studies by clinical area they supported. We found that seven studies (41%) were used for several clinical areas [12, 16, 18, 19, 25–27].

The major supported areas were management of chronic medical conditions or preventive care (n = 7, 41%) [11, 14–16, 22, 23, 27] and management of acute medical conditions (n = 7, 41%) [12, 16–19, 26, 27]. This was followed in frequency by surgical procedures [18, 20, 24], monitoring surgical trauma intensive care units (ICU) [19, 26], pharmacotherapy (example of drug safety, infection control, rational use of antibiotics) [12, 21, 25], diagnosis [18], laboratory test ordering [13], surveillance and operational control of hospital-acquired infections or multidrug resistant infections [12, 26].

3.5.4 Were outcomes measured?

In most studies outcomes were not measured (n = 10, 59%) or reported (n = 2, 12%). Two studies reported more than one type of patient outcome measured (algorithm evaluation, time spent, etc.) [21, 27], specific tests such as oxygenation of the blood, heartbeats, daily steps, etc. [19], wound healing and/or length of stay, and time spent [12, 14].

3.5.5 Clinical and usability outcomes

Clinical outcomes. Clinical care, clinical research and patient outcomes are components of decision making and decision support processes that affect clinical outcomes. All of the studies [11–27] reported at least one clinical outcome, and most of them reported several. Fourteen studies (82%) [11–13, 16, 18–27] reported potential clinical care outcomes, such as quality of healthcare delivery and patient outcomes [18, 22–26], compliance [11, 25], adequate antibiotic use [12], identifying patients with decompensating physiology via a visual aid [18], clinician performance on clinically relevant tasks [27], accuracy (i.e. the system facilitates doctors developing preventive strategies depending on the timely and accurate identification of the greatest perioperative complication risks for patients, while the system provides accurate information such as improved calculated risk score) [20, 26]. Others included determining healthcare provider confidence (i.e. making physicians more confident that they were not missing crucial information) [27], efficiency (how to quickly detect inappropriate treatment, or help provide better care and faster response to adverse events) [21, 26]. Two studies (12%) in addition to clinical care outcomes reported that their system could be used in a research setting [11, 13]. Nearly half of the studies (n = 8, 47%) reported patient outcomes [14, 15, 17, 19, 20, 22, 23, 26] such as patient safety [17, 20], reduced hospital stay [19, 22, 23], earlier detection of disease, adverse events [19, 26], and time spent for each patient state [14, 15].

Usability outcomes. This refers to whether the system that was developed is easy to use, cost efficient and satisfactory for the users. Only two studies did not report usability outcomes [16, 26]. Ten studies (59%) reported effectiveness of their systems, such as gaining more knowledge [12, 18, 21–25] and decreasing errors [13], effectiveness usage to estimate changes over time or to compare the estimated risks from one hospital to another [17], and optimizing and planning resources [13]. Six studies (35%) reported efficiency outcomes, such as low costs [17, 18] and time needed on clinically relevant tasks [11, 19, 20, 26]. Almost 30% of the studies (n = 5) included satisfaction outcomes, such as satisfaction with system usage [23, 27], visual validity (i.e. real time and interactive visualization on physician smartphone applications) [14, 22, 23], improvement and user friendliness [16].

3.5.6 Outcomes effect

Only six studies (35%) included quantitative measures that could validate the outcome changes in their studies [12, 14, 19, 21, 26, 27].

One study [12] reported that their system increased predictive power for patient admissions (ICU) and 30% success in predicting an event 7 days before it occurs. This study reported that when the system was used, they found decreasing negative patient outcomes (death, disease, adverse reactions, infections)—50% of patient deaths were predicted within 7 days before the event occurred. Ninety-five percent of all decisions (an increase from 30%) were based on information coming from the system [12]. They concluded that monitoring antibiotic use in real-time, either from an institutional or individual perspective, immediately generated targeted interventions that led to more adequate antibiotic use.

Another study [14] reported that both doctors and normal users are getting more and more familiar with the system as a function of "disease numbers" (comorbidity) increases. A person with four diseases understands visualization outputs three times more quickly than a person with only one disease (30 s vs. 90 s). User satisfaction increases as well since they can now understand disease diagnosis results diagrams faster (from 6 (for patient with 1 disease) to near 10 (for patient with 4 diseases) on a scale of 0–10.

In another study, the rate of septic shock in the Surgical and Trauma Intensive Care Unit (STICU) decreased by more than half after the display of the system monitor was made available to the STICU ($p < 0.05$). These results remained statistically significant even after adjusting for other control variables. The rates of respiratory failure, hemorrhage and mortality did not change significantly in either unit when comparing the periods before and after monitor display [19].

Time to detection of an inappropriate treatment decreased when using an algorithm (sorted and ordered sequences) developed for one system [21]. The study also reported that the algorithm is a very good classifier when compared with a pharmacovigilance expert (gold standard review). Another study [27] reported a non-statistically significant difference in time on clinically relevant tasks, but many others reported improved potential outcomes without any quantitative measures.

Fourteen studies (82.4%) mentioned the potential gain in knowledge for clinical decision support [11, 13, 14, 17–27], eight studies (47%) reported a potential to decrease negative patient outcomes (death, disease, adverse reactions, infections) [12, 16, 18–20, 24–26], seven studies (41%) reported improved clinical decisions based on information [12–15, 21, 23, 25]. Six studies (35%) mentioned improved/increased patient outcomes (e.g. blood sugar, decreased length of stay, saved time) [11, 16, 18, 23, 24, 26]. Three studies (18%) reported that system implementation will decrease cost of care [22, 23, 26], and one study (6%) reported increased predictive power due to system use [12].

3.6 PICOS classification: part 5: study design

The subcategories of the PICOS classification of the study design are presented in **Table 5**. Three subcategories were identified that could classify the study design, including: (1) analytics and descriptive study design, (2) study design score and (3) whether the system was a prototype or actually used in practice. Thirteen

PICOS subcategory		Description	All studies	All studies, %
STUDY DESIGN	Analytics	Analytic; Case-Crossover	1	5.9
		Analytic; Experimental;	3	17.6
		Analytic; Observational	1	5.9
	Descriptive	Qualitative	13	76.5
		Qualitative; Survey	1	5.9
		User-centered, iterative design	1	5.9
STUDY DESIGN SCORE		1 (qualitative design)	10	58.8
		2 (quantitative descriptive design)	1	5.9
		3 (mixed qualitative and quantitative descriptive)	6	35.3
PRACTICE OR PROTOTYPE		Practice (used in practice)	4	23.5
		Prototype (real data)	13	76.5

Table 5.
PICOS classification of all publications: Part 5: study design.

studies (77%) were identified as descriptive (qualitative) studies, although 10 (59%) of them were identified only as qualitative designs [11, 13, 16, 18, 20, 22–26], three were identified as mixed qualitative and quantitative descriptive [12, 14, 19], one was identified as descriptive qualitative with survey [15] and one was descriptive with user-centered, iterative design [27]. Five studies (29%) used analytics designs [12, 14, 17, 19, 21].

Most of the studies reviewed (n = 13, 77%) were prototypes but with results based on real data. Only four of the studies reported systems (23%) actually used in practice.

4. Conclusion

To provide effective patient-centered healthcare, it is essential to manage and analyze huge amounts of data. In the past decade, the variety and volume of health data sources have both increased dramatically, making traditional data management and analysis tools insufficient. Big data has emerged as a response to the growing need for health organizations to have new tools capable of processing massive amounts and varieties of healthcare data [30]. A major advantage of big data techniques is the use of advanced analysis techniques such as predictive analytics to improve clinical care, quality of care and patient outcomes.

This systematic review identified 17 studies with different visualization types and user intents, with a wide variety of data collection methods, big data platforms and tools, clinical decision support purposes to understand and synthesize existing approaches of big data knowledge visualization for clinical decision support. The results of this review emphasize the use of common types of big data knowledge visualization, patterns of big data analytics methods and classification of outcomes for clinical decision support.

The study demonstrated big differences in terms of visualization techniques used, user intents, big data tool implementations and outcome effects. Most studies reported only potential effectiveness from using knowledge visualization in clinical setting. This included gaining more knowledge for clinical decision support and improved clinical decision making based on better and more timely information, decreasing negative patient outcomes (i.e. death, disease, adverse reactions, infections) and improving patient outcomes (i.e. blood sugar, decreased length of stay and time saving), increasing predictive power of adverse events, and decreasing cost of care. Much more research is needed on implementing different techniques for big data knowledge visualization and evaluating the resulting outcomes from clinical decision support. Additional study is also needed to provide solid evidence that clinical outcomes can be improved through clinical decision support through big data knowledge visualization.

5. Limitations

Our study has three limitations. First, we only searched publications in English, and thus did not capture studies published in other languages. We also did not include commercial applications/systems which are used for clinical decision support and which may be using advanced techniques for knowledge visualization support. Lastly, papers on big data knowledge visualization but not implemented on big data platforms/tools were excluded from our review. Additional knowledge to understand big data knowledge visualization for clinical decision support could be possible through a review of such systems.

Author details

Mehrdad Roham, Anait R. Gabrielyan and Norm Archer*
DeGroote Business School, McMaster University, Hamilton, ON, Canada

*Address all correspondence to: rohamm@mcmaster.ca

IntechOpen

© 2019 The Author(s). Licensee IntechOpen. This chapter is distributed under the terms of the Creative Commons Attribution License (http://creativecommons.org/licenses/by/3.0), which permits unrestricted use, distribution, and reproduction in any medium, provided the original work is properly cited.

References

[1] Greenes RA. Definition, scope, and challenges. In: Clinical Decision Support. Academic Press; 2007. pp. 3-29

[2] Munzner T. Visualization Design and Analysis: Abstractions, Principles, and Methods [Internet]. 2012. Available from: http://web.cse.ohio-state.edu/~machiraju.1/teaching/CSE5544/ClassLectures/PDF-old/book.120803.pdf

[3] Stadler JG, Donlon K, Siewert JD, Franken T, Lewis NE. Improving the efficiency and ease of healthcare analysis through use of data visualization dashboards. Big Data. 2016;**4**(2):129-135

[4] Moher D, Liberati A, Tetzlaff J, Altman DG, Altman D, Antes G, et al. Preferred reporting items for systematic reviews and meta-analyses: The PRISMA statement (Chinese edition). PLoS Medicine. 2009;**6**(7):e1000097

[5] Liberati A, Altman DG, Tetzlaff J, Mulrow C, Gøtzsche PC, Ioannidis JPA, et al. The PRISMA statement for reporting systematic reviews and meta-analyses of studies that evaluate health care interventions: Explanation and elaboration. PLoS Medicine. 2009;**6**(7):e1000100

[6] Higgins J, Green S, editors. Cochrane Handbook for Systematic Reviews of Interventions Version 5.1.0. Cochrane Collaboration; 2011

[7] Wu DTY, Chen AT, Manning JD, Levy-fix G, Backonja U, Borland D, et al. Review. Evaluating visual analytics for health informatics applications: A systematic review from the American medical informatics association visual analytics working group task force on evaluation. Journal of the American Medical Informatics Association. 2019;**26**(February):314-323

[8] Rind BA, Wang TD, Aigner W, Miksch S, Wongsuphasawat K, Plaisant C, et al. Interactive information visualization to explore and query electronic health records and ben Shneiderman. Foundations and Trends® in Human-Computer Interaction. 2013;**5**(3):207-298

[9] Yi JS, Kang Y, Stasko JT, Jacko JA. Interaction taxonomy. IEEE Transactions on Visualization and Computer Graphics. 2007;**13**(6):1224-1231

[10] Hong L, Luo M, Wang R, Lu P, Wei Lu LL. Big data in health care: Applications and challenges. Data and Information Management. 2018;**2**(3):175-197

[11] Chen H, Compton S, Hsiao O. DiabeticLink: A health big data system for patient empowerment and personalized healthcare. Lecture Notes in Computer Science (including Subser Lect Notes Artif Intell Lect Notes Bioinformatics). 2013;**8040 LNCS**:71-83

[12] Feng Z, Bhat RR, Yuan X, Freeman D, Baslanti T, Bihorac A, et al. Intelligent perioperative system: Towards real-time big data analytics in surgery risk assessment. In: Proc - 2017 IEEE 15th Int Conf Dependable, Auton Secur Comput 2017 IEEE 15th Int Conf Pervasive Intell Comput 2017 IEEE 3rd Int Conf Big Data Intell Compu. Vol. 2018-Jan. 2018. pp. 1254-1259

[13] Ledieu T, Bouzille G, Plaisant C, Thiessard F, Polard E, Cuggia M. Mining clinical big data for drug safety: Detecting inadequate treatment with a DNA sequence alignment algorithm. AMIA Annual Symposium Proceedings. 2018;**2018**:1368-1376

[14] Serhani MA, El Menshawy M, Benharref A, Harous S, Navaz AN. New

algorithms for processing time-series big EEG data within mobile health monitoring systems. Computer Methods and Programs in Biomedicine. 2017;**149**(2017):79-94

[15] Serhani MA, El Menshawy M, Benharref A. SME2EM: Smart mobile end-to-end monitoring architecture for life-long diseases. Computers in Biology and Medicine. 2016;**68**:137-154

[16] Li P, Yates SN, Lovely JK, Larson DW. Patient-like-mine: A real time, visual analytics tool for clinical decision support. In: Proc - 2015 IEEE Int Conf Big Data. 2015. pp. 2865-2867

[17] Morales A, Cánovas-Segura B, Campos M, Juarez JM, Palacios F. Proposal of a big data platform for intelligent antibiotic surveillance in a hospital. In: Oscar L, Gámez JA, Barrenechea E, Troncoso A, Galar M, Quintián H, et al., editors. Advances in Artificial Intelligence. Cham: Springer International Publishing; 2016. pp. 261-270

[18] Baljak V, Ljubovic A, Michel J, Montgomery M, Salaway R. A scalable realtime analytics pipeline and storage architecture for physiological monitoring big data. Smart Healing. 2018;**9-10**:275-286

[19] Hirsch JS, Tanenbaum JS, Gorman SL, Liu C, Schmitz E, Hashorva D, et al. HARVEST, a longitudinal patient record summarizer. Journal of the American Medical Informatics Association. 2015;**22**(2):263-274

[20] Almeida JP. A disruptive big data approach to leverage the efficiency in management and clinical decision support in a hospital. Porto Biomedical Journal. 2016;**1**(1):40-42

[21] Li D, Park HW, Batbaatar E. In: Nguyen N, Hoang D, Hong TP, Pham H, Trawiński B, editors. Intelligent Information and Database Systems. Vol. 10751. 2018. pp. 684-693

[22] Galletta A, Carnevale L, Bramanti A, Fazio M. An innovative methodology for big data visualization for telemedicine. IEEE Trans Ind Informatics. 2019;**15**(1):490-497

[23] Suresh S. Big data and predictive analytics: Applications in the care of children. Pediatric Clinics of North America. 2016;**63**(2):357-366

[24] Caron A, Chazard E, Muller J, Perichon R, Ferret L, Koutkias V, et al. IT-CARES: An interactive tool for case-crossover analyses of electronic medical records for patient safety. Journal of the American Medical Informatics Association. 2017;**24**(2):323-330

[25] Badgeley MA, Shameer K, Glicksberg BS, Tomlinson MS, Levin MA, McCormick PJ, et al. EHDViz: Clinical dashboard development using open-source technologies. BMJ Open. 2016;**6**(3):1-11

[26] Abusharekh A, Stewart SA, Hashemian N, Abidi SSR. H-DRIVE: A big health data analytics platform for evidence-informed decision making. Proc - 2015 IEEE Int Congr Big Data. 2015; (c):416-423.

[27] Ruminski CM, Clark MT, Lake DE, Kitzmiller RR, Keim-Malpass J, Robertson MP, et al. Impact of predictive analytics based on continuous cardiorespiratory monitoring in a surgical and trauma intensive care unit. Journal of Clinical Monitoring and Computing. 2019;**33**:703

[28] Aigner W, Miksch S, Schumann H, Tominski C. Visualization of Time-Oriented Data. Human-Computer Interaction. Springer-Verlag London Limited; 2011

[29] von Landesberger T, Fiebig S, Bremm S, Kuijper A, Fellner DW. Interaction taxonomy for tracking of user actions in visual analytics applications. In: Huang W, editor. Handbook of Human Centric Visualization. New York, NY: Springer New York; 2014. pp. 653-670

[30] Alonso SG, de la Torre Díez I, Rodrigues JJPC, Hamrioui S, López-Coronado M. A systematic review of techniques and sources of big data in the healthcare sector. Journal of Medical Systems. 2017;**41**(11)

Chapter 8

WASPSS: A Clinical Decision Support System for Antimicrobial Stewardship

Bernardo Cánovas Segura, Antonio Morales, Jose M. Juarez, Manuel Campos and Francisco Palacios

Abstract

The increase of infections caused by resistant bacteria has become one of the major health-care problems worldwide. The creation of multidisciplinary teams dedicated to the implementation of antimicrobial stewardship programmes (ASPs) is encouraged by all clinical institutions to cope with this problem. In this chapter, we describe the Wise Antimicrobial Stewardship Program Support System (WASPSS), a CDSS focused on providing support for ASP teams. WASPSS gathers the required information from other hospital systems in order to provide decision support in antimicrobial stewardship from both patient-centered and global perspectives. To achieve this, it combines business intelligence techniques with a rule-based inference engine to integrate the data and knowledge required in this scenario. The system provides functions such as alerts, recommendations, antimicrobial prescription support and global surveillance. Furthermore, it includes experimental modules for improving the adoption of clinical guidelines and applying prediction models related with antimicrobial resistance. All these functionalities are provided through a multi-user web interface, personalized for each role of the ASP team.

Keywords: antimicrobial stewardship, antimicrobial resistance, infection management, rule-based systems, data and knowledge integration, clinical practice guidelines

1. Introduction

Antibiotics have been one of the most significant discoveries in medicine, to the point that some researches talk about pre-antibiotic and post-antibiotic eras in clinical practice due to their repercussion in the treatment of infectious diseases [1]. However, bacteria are able to develop resistance against antibiotics when they are exposed to them for a long period of time. Indeed, in a short time after the widespread usage of a novel antibiotic, new strains of bacteria resistant to it have appeared [2]. The problem is so severe that international health organizations claim that "... a post-antibiotic era -in which common infections and minor injures can kill- is a very real possibility for the 21st century" [3].

It has been recognized by global health organizations that one of the main causes of this problem, also known as *antimicrobial resistance*, is the overuse of antibiotics. For this reason, they are encouraging the adoption of *antimicrobial stewardship*

IntechOpen

programmes (ASPs) [4–7], in order to develop specific actuations and protocols to improve the antimicrobial usage and limit the rise of antimicrobial resistance. These programs include recommendations about all the actions related to the use of antimicrobials in clinical practice, such as the appropriateness of a particular antibiotic for an infection, its dosage, the route of administration or the duration of the therapy [4].

Due to the complexity of this problem, one of the recommendations for the hospital setting is to constitute a multidisciplinary team, called the *antimicrobial stewardship programme team (ASP team)*. This team should be composed of specialists from different clinical areas such as physicians, epidemiologists, pharmacists, microbiologists and managers. The coordination of efforts obtained thanks to the diversity of the ASP team members is seen as fundamental in order to achieve an improvement in the rational use of antimicrobials within the institution.

First experiences in the implementation of ASP teams have obtained limited but satisfactory results regarding the usage of antimicrobials [8, 9]. A well-known disadvantage of the ASP methodology is the amount of time required by ASP members to review alerts and documentation [10]. Therefore, these studies also state the need for computerized tools to help with these complex tasks. The use of clinical decision support systems (CDSSs) can be a key factor in improving the results of ASP teams, taking into account the multi-user perspective of the problem, the need for data and knowledge integration from different sources, and the requirement to provide support both for a particular patient and for the whole institution in a coordinated manner. In this chapter, we perform an overview of different studies related with decision support in antimicrobial resistance and perform a detailed description of the *Wise Antimicrobial Stewardship Program Support System (WASPSS)*, a CDSS focused on ASP teams.

2. Decision support in the context of antimicrobial resistance

Infectious diseases were one of first clinical topics related with decision support systems. One of these first systems was MYCIN [11], which relied on production rules derived from discussions with clinical experts to provide suggestions about the diagnosis and appropriate management of infected patients. Although the system was never used clinically, it was a relevant reference for the research and development of CDSSs during the 1980s [12].

Another relevant work was the HELP system [13], which provided alerts, reports and suggestions obtained from the data available in clinical records. With additional epidemiologic data and expert knowledge, it was used to provide recommendations about antibiotic treatments and therapies [14].

The infections acquired within clinical institutions (i.e., nosocomial infections) are commonly caused by bacteria resistant to antibiotics and, therefore, harder to treat. The relevance of these infections led researchers to focus on this problem. The GermWatcher expert system [15, 16] is capable of evaluating the results of cultures with the aim of detecting nosocomial infections. GermWatcher uses a rule engine whose knowledge base is based on the guidelines of the Nosocomial Infection Surveillance System from the Centers for Disease Control. Thanks to them, it is capable of classifying the alert level of a microorganism and deciding whether or not to report it as a nosocomial infection.

The Mercurio system [17] is also focused on the detection and monitoring of nosocomial infections. It was intended for different kinds of users, such as laboratory physicians, clinicians and epidemiologists, and included knowledge from several sources, such as antibiotic hierarchical definitions and international guidelines for microbiological laboratories. It is capable of checking the susceptibility tests in order to ensure that they have been performed according to the guidelines, differentiating among possible strains of bacteria, and warning about possible outbreaks of a particular strain. Furthermore, association rules are used to identify local resistance patterns that are not covered by the standard guidelines.

Another example focused on this problem is the HASIS information system [18] that implements the guidelines for hospital-acquired infections published by the Centers for Disease Control and Prevention and includes algorithms for the detection of suspicious cases. It employs a service-oriented architecture as a basis on which to integrate the surveillance data required for this task.

However, the rise and spread of multidrug-resistant bacteria has forced the research community to tackle the problem of nosocomial infections from the broader perspective of antimicrobial stewardship.

The DebugIT (Detecting and Eliminating Bacteria UsinG Information Technology) European project [19] was developed to gather information about antimicrobial resistance from heterogeneous sources [20]. It uses semantic web technologies to structure data and is capable of performing data analysis on it in order to provide decision support [21].

From yet another point of view, the TREAT system [22] uses causal probabilistic networks to propose an antibiotic treatment when the infectious agent is still unknown, based on the local epidemiological data and clinical observations such as the site of infection, symptoms and background disorders. This signifies that the spectrum of the treatments can be narrower, and less antimicrobial resistance is, therefore, developed.

Other proposals are focused on intensive care units (ICUs), since they are the hospital wards with the highest number of nosocomial infections and multi-resistant bacteria.

For example, the objective of the MoniICU system [23] is to identify and monitor nosocomial infections in ICUs. It uses production rules defined by using ARDEN syntax, an HL7 standard oriented toward sharing medical knowledge. Furthermore, it includes a fuzzy abstraction module for the definition of nosocomial infections.

Another example is the COSARA platform [24], which is focused on infection surveillance in ICUs. It provides functionalities for the automatic integration of clinical data and clinical decision support and alerts to alarming trends, among others.

Recently, some relevant works have been finally focused on supporting ASP teams in order to assess in the use of antibiotics by hospitals. The Antimicrobial Prescription Surveillance System [25] is focused on identifying potentially inappropriate antimicrobial prescriptions and reporting them to pharmacists. It has a knowledge base with contraindications regarding drug–drug interactions, drug-bug mismatches and maximum daily dose, among others. Furthermore, the system includes a learning algorithm with which to evaluate the feedback regarding the launched alerts and reduce the number of those that are erroneous or clinically irrelevant.

In Evans et al. [26], a framework of medical informatics tools is proposed in order to provide ASP teams with support. It automatically generates spreadsheets containing the antibiotics that are used daily and the parameters available to decide the antimicrobial therapy for specific patients. It additionally sends e-mail and SMS alerts to ASP members when timely-critical laboratory results are available, such as positive blood or cerebrospinal fluid cultures. Finally, it generates different reports based on the National Healthcare Safety Network specifications.

The HAITooL system [27] is also focused on ASP teams. It monitors antibiotic usage, rates antibiotic-resistant bacteria and allows early identification of outbreaks. It integrates evidence-based algorithms with which to support proper antibiotic prescription.

And a final example is the Wise Antimicrobial Stewardship Program Support System (WASPSS) [10]. WASPSS is focused on ASP team support and gathers information for multiple hospital information systems in order to provide a unified decision support for typical ASP tasks. It is the CDSS explained in detail in this chapter.

3. The WASPSS project

The University Hospital of Getafe (UHG) is a medium-size hospital (approximately 450 beds), which is located in Madrid, Spain. It has units covering most medical specialities, including a burns unit, although there are no cardiac surgery or transplant units. In 2014, the UHG set up an antibiotic stewardship programme denominated as "program for the multidisciplinary care in the assessment and control of the antimicrobial therapy" (PAMACTA) [10]. The PAMACTA team is composed of members from different specialities, including pharmacists, microbiologists, surgeons, internists, intensivists and infection preventionists. This team has been formed to address two organizational proposals: (a) to include a representative of each hospital service, or at least those services with a higher use of antibiotics, and (b) to involve all the physicians as part of the ASP. The intention of these two proposals is to reduce the time spent on distributing the task among departments and the integration of individual clinical expertise with the best available external clinical evidence, a basic principle of evidence-based medicine [28].

The *Wise Antibiotic Stewardship Program Support System* (WASPSS) platform [10, 29] is a CDSS focused on ASPs and infectious disease management. It was developed by the University of Murcia in collaboration with UHG at the same time as the PAMACTA team was created, which provided the opportunity to focus on the current needs of an ASP team starting from scratch. WASPSS is currently in the production stage and it is used daily by the PAMACTA team. Furthermore, it is being piloted in other seven public hospitals in Spain.

4. System architecture overview

An overview of the WASPSS software architecture is shown in **Figure 1**. The system is capable of obtaining information from multiple hospital information systems, which is a key factor to provide a proper support to the ASP team. The hospital systems and some examples of data collected by WASPSS are the following:

- Pharmacy systems: the dispensations or administrations of antimicrobials

- Microbiology laboratory: the results of cultures, the microorganisms found, and the resistances or susceptibilities found in the laboratory

- Clinical tests laboratory: white-cell count, creatinine levels and other infection-related tests

- Electronic health records (EHR): data related to patient, such as previous stays, current ward, and stays at ICU.

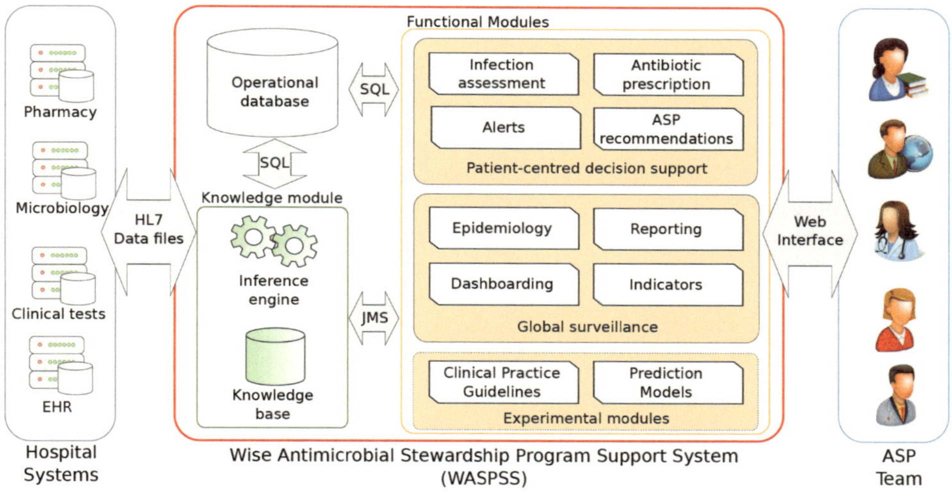

Figure 1.
Overview of the WASPSS platform and its different modules.

To perform data integration, a *Health Level 7* (*HL7*) interface engine has been included. HL7 is a widely accepted set of standards for interoperability between health care organizations. HL7 provides messaging for exchanging, sharing and retrieving electronic health information between medical applications in near real time. Most HIS vendors adhere to these standards when developing application interfaces to exchange patient data. Additionally, WASPSS also supports the batch-loading of data files for those cases in which the HL7 interface is not available. Furthermore, a *Java Message Service* server is also used for the communication between WASPSS modules.

The data collected from hospital systems are filtered, structured and stored into an operational database by using extract-transform-load processes. This database acts as a centralized data hub for all the WASPSS modules.

WASPSS uses artificial intelligence techniques to provide proper support for ASP teams. In particular, WASPSS includes a knowledge module to incorporate clinical literature and daily practice knowledge [30–32]. To this end, the module implements a rule-based reasoning architecture composed of a knowledge base and a rule-based engine. The knowledge base contains production rules, ontologies and other business process models related with antimicrobial stewardship. The rule-based engine can make use of both the knowledge base and the data collected from the hospital to perform abstractions, raise alerts or evaluate processes, and its results can be stored back into the database or communicated through JMS to the other WASPSS modules.

Finally, the system includes a web-based interface that offers a different front-end for each user role of the ASP team, facilitating its usage for each clinician involved with antimicrobial stewardship within the institution. In the next sections, we describe in detail the capabilities of WASPSS to provide decision support for tasks related with both particular patients and the whole clinical organization.

5. Patient-centered decision support

The capability of WASPSS to aggregate information from different hospital systems allows to provide comprehensive decision support for a particular patient. This is especially useful in antibiotic prescription and patient-related alerts, as explained next.

5.1 Antibiotic prescription

The selection of the most appropriate antibiotic treatment is a key decision both to improve the patient's health and to reduce the risk of antimicrobial resistance for the community. However, it usually occurs that the microorganism responsible for the infection has not yet been determined when the clinician must decide the antibiotic therapy to use. In these situations, clinicians must use all the available information about the patient and the infection (possible focus, previous infections, etc.) along with the information regarding the common pathogens found in the hospital and their resistance patterns, which is called the *local cumulative antibiogram*. After deciding this initial therapy, known as *empiric therapy*, clinicians can adjust, suspend or incorporate antibiotics when the infecting microorganism is found and analyzed, starting then a *targeted therapy*. However, the development of a local cumulative antibiogram is a time-consuming task that requires gathering information about the microorganisms found within the institution, and therefore, it is usually generated yearly.

The *antibiotic prescription module* of WASPSS assists physicians in the prescription of appropriate empiric or targeted antibiotic treatments (**Figure 2**). Thanks to the data collected from the microbiology system, WASPSS can calculate the cumulative antibiograms instantly. Furthermore, it can use data from any period and stratify them attending to different criteria in order to obtain, for example, the most effective antibiotic for blood infections in the ICU ward during the last year.

The efficacy of each antibiotic is computed under those criteria, from 1 (less effective) to 100 (fully effective), based on the number needed to fail measure [33]. Finally, a list with the available antibiotics ranked by efficacy and confidence interval is proposed to the physician. The tool shows additional notes about each option, such as whether a restricted use of the antibiotic is recommended or if it can be administered orally. Furthermore, the tool can present the list of most common microorganisms found under the search criteria, along with their susceptibilities to antimicrobials. A graphical view of the results is also available through a bipartite model, which represents the relationships between microorganisms and antibiotics by means of channels of different width [34]. With these tools, physicians can take a more informed decision related with both empiric and targeted antimicrobial therapies.

5.2 Alerts, recommendations and assessment of infections

One of the common decision support tasks from CDSSs is to alert clinicians when certain events occur. In case of the antimicrobial stewardship scenario, typical alerts are related with the detection of bacteria resistant to multiple antibiotics, the results of tests that indicate severe infections, the prescription of restricted antibiotics or the opportunities to change the route of administration of an antibiotic to a less aggressive route for a patient.

WASPSS includes a pre-defined set of these alerts in the form of production rules within its knowledge base. Furthermore, as shown in **Figure 3**, clinicians may use the web-based interface to perform detailed queries that can also be stored as new alerts. If that is the case, the query is translated into production rules, stored in the knowledge base and executed daily. Each new case found will be notified then as any other alert automatically.

One recurrent problem is CDSSs is the *alarm fatigue*, that is, users tend to ignore all alerts when too many of them are launched [35]. In order to cope with this problem, WASPSS allows to define alerts with three different levels of severity. Furthermore, alerts can be restricted to specific user profiles. By this way, each user

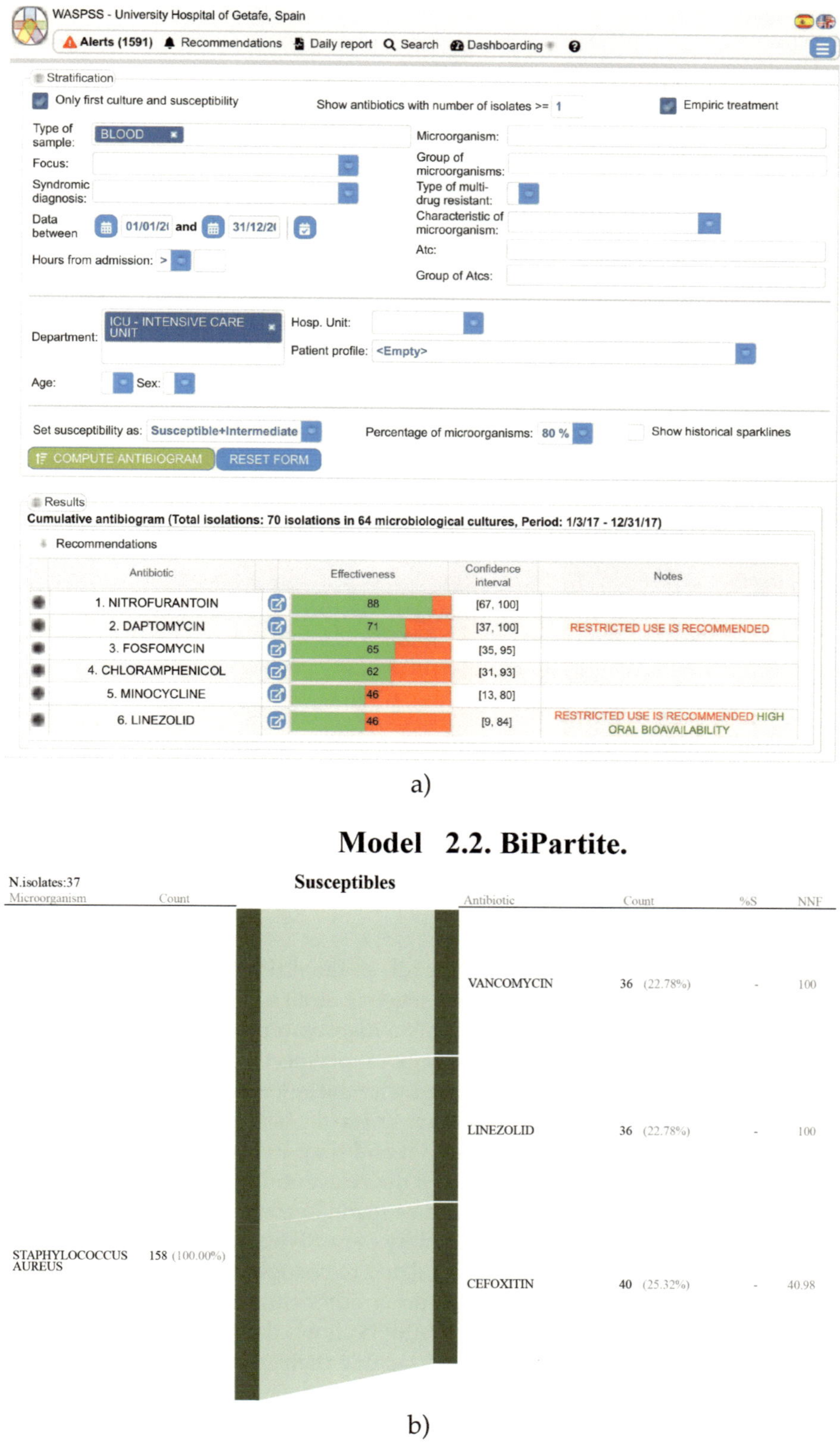

Figure 2.
Screenshot of the antibiotic prescription module. Given a search criteria, a rank of most effective antimicrobials is provided based on the local cumulative antibiogram (a). A graphical bipartite model is also available in order to show relationships between antibiotics and microorganisms (b). The antimicrobial efficacy data shown in this picture are fictitious.

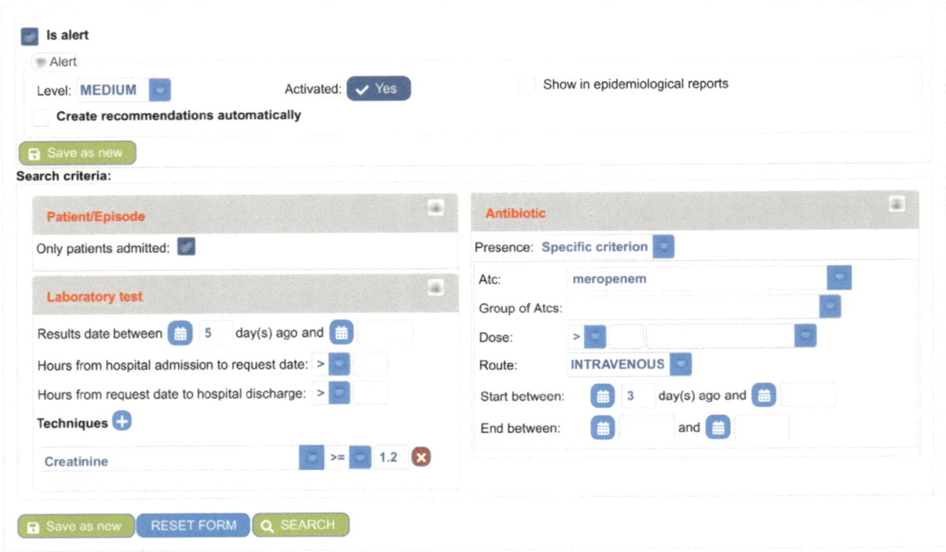


```
rule "Meropenem-Indication␣of␣dose␣adjustment␣based␣on␣renal␣function"
when
  $c: Clock()
  $p: Patient(isAdmitted == true)
  $a: Antibiotic(patient==$p, atcCode == "J01DH05", // Meropenem
      route == "IV", startDate >= substract_days($c.now, 3, "days"))
  $l: LaboratoryTest(patient == $p,
      requestDate >= substract_days($c.now, 5, "days"))
  and exists (
    TechniqueResult(labTest == $l, tech == "Creatinine", result >= 1.2)
  )
then
  insert (new Alert(drools.getRule(), "MEDIUM", $p, $a, $l))
end
```

Figure 3.
Screenshot of the alerts module. Clinicians can build detailed queries with a user-friendly interface. Those queries considered as relevant can be automatically translated into production rules and stored as new alerts in the knowledge base.

receives only those alerts relevant to their role in the ASP team, and they can decide whether to revise only those with higher severity or all of them.

To manage each particular alert, WASPSS displays a patient-centered timeline view (**Figure 4**). This view provides a temporal perspective of all the data recovered from hospital systems that are related with antimicrobial stewardship, such as treatments, cultures, clinical tests and stays in wards. When an alert is fired, it is linked with the clinical events that caused it and they are highlighted in this view. By this way, the ASP team can evaluate all the relevant data regarding a patient when deciding which clinical action must be made in response to each alert.

Most of the clinical actions undertaken by the ASP team consist of performing recommendations to the physician staff related to changes in the antibiotic therapy of a particular patient, or to suggest cultures or other clinical tests whose results can improve the treatment of an infection. WASPSS allows the ASP team to create those recommendations for a specific patient, attaching their reasons and the suggested actions. Physicians can then access these recommendations by using the WASPSS platform. Optionally, these recommendations can be sent through the HL7 interface to other systems in order to facilitate the daily hospital workflow.

Alerts can also generate automatically informed recommendations that only need to be validated by the ASP team in order to be communicated. For example, WASPSS can detect that an antibiotic that is being administered by the intravenous route for many days can also be administered orally, which is less aggressive for the

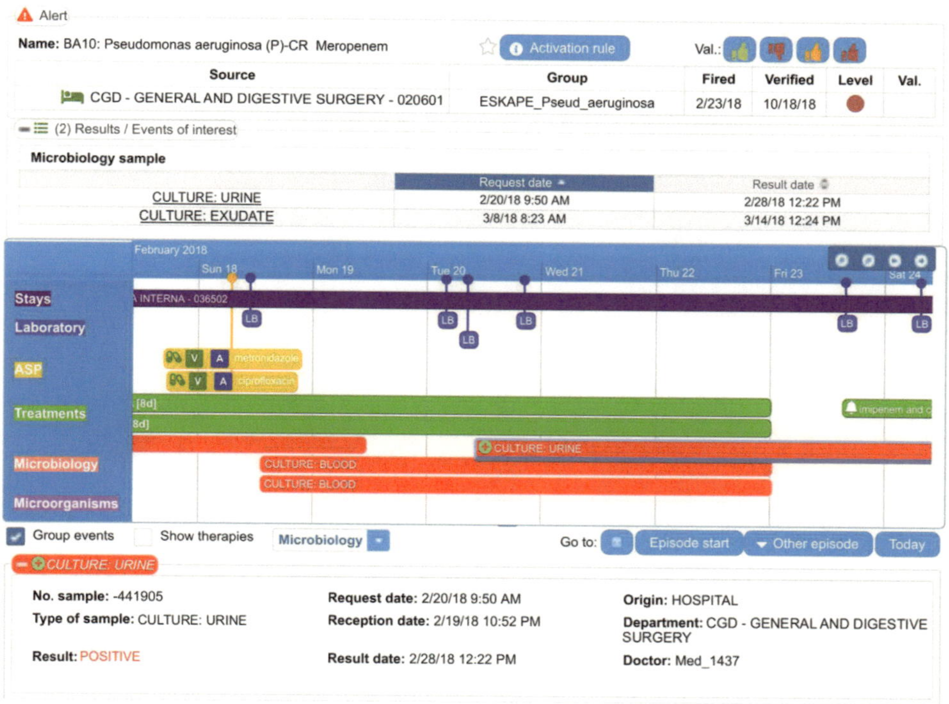

Figure 4.
Screenshot of the timeline view with the details of the alert and all the patient's clinical events. The patient's data shown in this picture are fictitious.

patient. Then, an alert is raised with a recommendation completed by the system, which includes the antibiotic, the suggestion of changing its administration route, and also the conditions that must be checked before undertaking this action, such as that the patient has no digestive problems that contraindicate the ingest of antibiotics.

WASPSS also facilitates the assessment of the infection for a particular patient. The patient-centered view includes the relevant data obtained from the EHR, along with the results from the microbiology tests and the rest of the clinical tests performed to the patient. The visualization of all these data in a clear and organized way facilitates the evaluation of the patient's infection by clinicians.

6. Institutional decision support

Along with the patient-centered perspective, a broader vision is required in order to perform a proper antimicrobial stewardship within the institution. The monitoring of both clinical and process outcomes is important for proposing new strategic actions, and also for removing measures or policies that are not having any real impact on patient safety, economy or antibiotic resistance.

Global surveillance and monitoring in WASPSS is achieved by four modules. First, the epidemiology module (**Figure 5a**) visualizes the evolution of statistical measures such as prevalence and incidence of microorganisms, antibiotics, microbiological sample types and alerts.

Second, the dashboarding module (**Figure 5b**) provides interactive charts that summarize global measures related to antibiograms, alerts and ASP recommendations over a specified time interval.

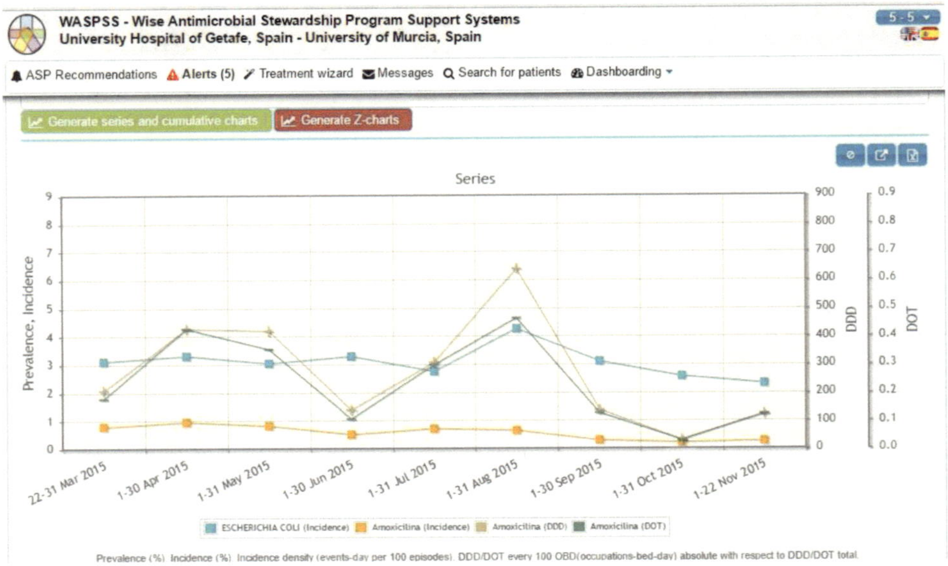

a)

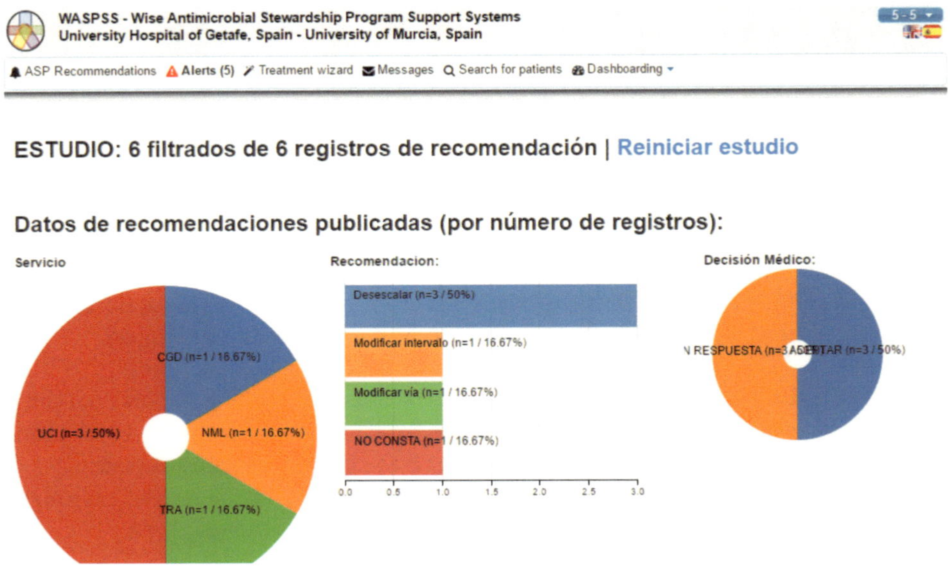

b)

Figure 5.
Global surveillance support in WASPSS: (a) epidemiology and (b) dashboarding modules. The data shown in this picture are fictitious.

Third, actionable reports are generated using the reporting module (**Figure 6a**). Currently, two kinds of parameterized reports are available: the first one lists all the antibiotics and microbiological tests of hospitalized patients during a specified period of time, grouped by department and sorted by bed number; the second one includes statistical information (prevalence, incidence, etc.) about all the microorganisms, antibiotics, sample types and alerts occurred over a specified time interval.

Last, the ASP indicator module computes several process indicators (**Figure 6b**) whose results are presented in two forms: (i) as a run chart showing the evolution of

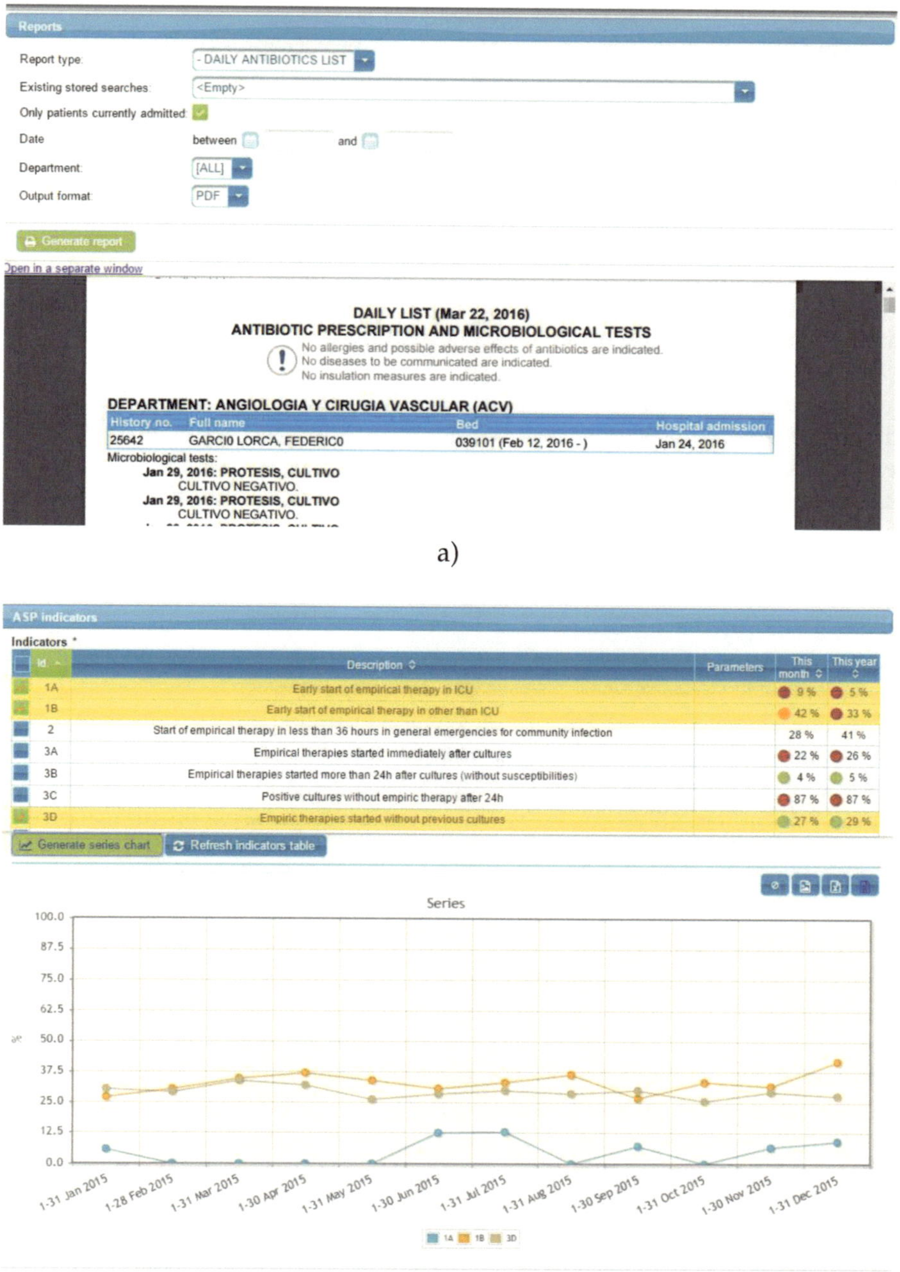

Figure 6.
Global surveillance support in WASPSS: (a) reporting and (b) ASP indicator modules. The data shown in this picture are fictitious.

the indicator over time and (ii) as a control table showing results of the current month and year, labeled with color codes indicating the goodness of the result.

7. Incorporation of clinical knowledge

WASPSS is also designed to incorporate different kinds of knowledge related with antimicrobial resistance [30].

The main source for the knowledge included is the expert rules from the EUropean Committee on Antimicrobial Susceptibility Testing (EUCAST) [36, 37]. These rules include the antibiotics to which each bacterial species is intrinsically resistant, those resistant patterns that are considered as exceptional and that should be re-checked to discard any problem on the laboratory tests, and resistance patterns that can be inferred from others found in laboratory.

WASPSS combines production rules with ontologies in order to incorporate the EUCAST rules in its knowledge base. Production rules are used to model most of the EUCAST knowledge, while ontologies are needed to model the hierarchical relationships of antibiotics and bacteria [31, 38].

This knowledge can be useful for many tasks such as the detection of incoherencies in laboratory results (e.g., bacteria that are found susceptible to an antibiotic to which they should be intrinsically resistant according to the EUCAST rules) and the detection of possible therapy failure because the infecting agent is found as resistant to all the antibiotics currently administered to the patient. In this last example, this knowledge has proved to be useful for increasing the number of cases detected and their clinical relevance [39].

8. Experimental features

The knowledge base and the inference engine provide opportunities for further knowledge-based expansions, incorporating knowledge from different sources. One of these sources can be the *Clinical Practice Guidelines* (*CPGs*), that is, widely accepted recommendations, processes and decision steps based on clinical evidence focused on improving the assistance of patients [40, 41]. Despite the fact that the use of CPGs has proved to improve clinical outcomes, they must be adapted to the particularities of each individual patient, which sometimes present a cumbersome problem for they use in daily practice [42].

WASPSS includes an experimental module to facilitate the visualization, adoption and evaluation of guidelines related with antimicrobial stewardship, focusing on the processes and decisions included in the guideline and those tasks that can be monitored thanks to the information gathered by the system [32]. An example of the graphical interface of this module is shown in **Figure** 7. The processes included in the guideline must be modeled by using the Business Process Model Notation (BPMN) and the decision-related recommendations by using the Decision Model Notation (DMN). These models are stored within the knowledge base and can be used to graphically visualize the tasks and decisions contained in the guideline. Production rules are then used to evaluate the status of each relevant task of the guideline and provide an estimation of the tasks already finished, those on-going and also those that may have been omitted. Finally, in combination with the patient-centered timeline view, the next guideline tasks can be scheduled in a flexible way, allowing the adaptation of the guideline to the particularities of each patient.

Another experimental extension is the incorporation of prediction models within the knowledge base. WASPSS includes an experimental clinical prediction rules module that is capable of incorporating prediction models based on logistic regression and evaluating them for a particular patient. Logistic regression is one of the most used techniques for developing models in clinical practice and can be combined with other techniques to deal with common problems related with data mining in antimicrobial resistance, such as unbalanced datasets or concept drift [43].

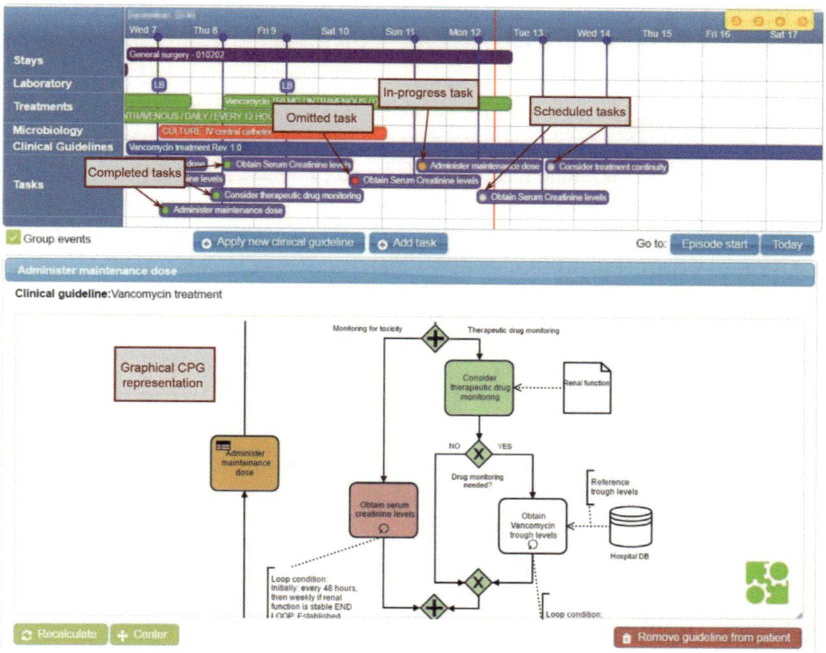

Figure 7.
Graphical interface for the CPG experimental module of WASPSS. The patient's data shown in this picture are fictitious.

9. Future work

When dealing with clinical data, it is usual to find uncertainties in test results, clinical guidelines or prediction models, especially due to missing patient data. As a future research line, we plan to detect these uncertainties as well as the data required to solve them when possible. Then, these data will be asked to the user and incorporated into the knowledge base to improve the results of the different WASPSS modules.

We consider that a grounded explanation of a recommendation is one of the key factors for the success of a CDSS. The methods and models used in WASPSS (production rules, ontologies, etc.) allow the traceability of any alert, decision or abstraction. Following this idea, we are studying the incorporation of explainable machine learning methods to improve the justifications of the results of the prediction models.

The use of WASPSS in several hospitals offers us the opportunity to combine efforts among different ASP teams to improve the global outcomes in antimicrobial stewardship. On the other hand, it raises the problems of the interchange of knowledge among hospitals [31] and the need for dealing with a huge amount of data, which may require the adaptation of WASPSS to a big data environment [44].

Other future changes may be taken into consideration as new technologies are adopted by the hospitals using WASPSS. For example, the Fast Healthcare Interoperability Resources (FHIR) protocol has become very popular in last years and its incorporation into WASPSS may be considered in the medium term.

10. Conclusions

CDSSs have been widely used to assist physicians when dealing with infectious diseases. However, the need for coordinated efforts against the rise of antimicrobial resistance urges them to provide new functionalities.

WASPSS is our proposal for a CDSS focused on the assistance of ASP teams in the hospital environment. It combines techniques from business intelligence and artificial intelligence to provide an integrated perspective for antimicrobial stewardship.

On the one hand, WASPSS collects data from multiple hospital information systems and incorporates knowledge in the form of alerts and expert EUCAST rules. It is also capable of incorporating knowledge from CPGs and prediction models related with antimicrobial resistance.

On the other hand, WASPSS provides alerts and functionalities for antibiotic prescription, ASP recommendations and infection assessment through a patient-centered view in order to assist physicians when taking decisions concerning a particular patient, and global surveillance modules to provide support for strategic decisions related with epidemiology, global clinical outcomes and reporting.

In conclusion and according to our experience with WASPSS, a multi-user perspective, capabilities to integrate data and knowledge from different sources, and both patient-centered and institutional perspectives are key requisites for any CDSS focused on antimicrobial stewardship.

Acknowledgements

This work was partially funded by the SITSUS project (Ref: RTI2018-094832-B-I00), given by the Spanish Ministry of Science, Innovation and Universities (MCIU), the Spanish Agency for Research (AEI) and the European Fund for Regional Development (FEDER).

Conflict of interest

The authors declare no conflict of interest.

Author details

Bernardo Cánovas Segura*†, Antonio Morales†, Jose M. Juarez†, Manuel Campos† and Francisco Palacios†
Faculty of Computer Science, University of Murcia, Spain

*Address all correspondence to: bernardocs@um.es

† These authors are contributed equally.

IntechOpen

© 2020 The Author(s). Licensee IntechOpen. This chapter is distributed under the terms of the Creative Commons Attribution License (http://creativecommons.org/licenses/by/3.0), which permits unrestricted use, distribution, and reproduction in any medium, provided the original work is properly cited.

References

[1] Aminov RI. A brief history of the antibiotic era: Lessons learned and challenges for the future. Frontiers in Microbiology. 2010;**1**(134):1-7

[2] Clatworthy AE, Pierson E, Hung DT. Targeting virulence: A new paradigm for antimicrobial therapy. Nature Chemical Biology. 2007;**3**(9):541-548

[3] Antimicrobial Resistance: Global Report on Surveillance—2014 Summary. Geneva: World Health Organization; 2014. Available from: http://www.who.int/drugresistance/documents/surveillancereport/en/. [Accessed: 28 August 2018]

[4] Dellit TH, Owens RC, McGowan JE, Gerding DN, Weinstein RA, Burke JP, et al. Infectious Diseases Society of America and the Society for Healthcare Epidemiology of America guidelines for developing an institutional program to enhance antimicrobial stewardship. Clinical Infectious Diseases. 2007;**44**(2): 159-177

[5] Doron S, Davidson LE. Antimicrobial stewardship. Mayo Clinic Proceedings. 2011;**86**(11):1113-1123

[6] Nathan C, Cars O. Antibiotic resistance—Problems, progress, and prospects. New England Journal of Medicine. 2014;**371**(19):1761-1763

[7] Magill SS, Edwards JR, Bamberg W, Beldavs ZG, Dumyati G, Kainer MA, et al. Multistate point-prevalence survey of health care-associated infections. New England Journal of Medicine. 2014; **370**(13):1198-1208

[8] Schentag JJ, Ballow CH, Fritz AL, Paladino JA, Williams JD, Cumbo TJ, et al. Changes in antimicrobial agent usage resulting from interactions among clinical pharmacy, the infectious disease division, and the microbiology laboratory. Diagnostic Microbiology and Infectious Disease. 1993;**16**(3): 255-264

[9] Carling P, Fung T, Killion A, Terrin N, Barza M. Favorable impact of a multidisciplinary antibiotic management program conducted during 7 years. Infection Control & Hospital Epidemiology. 2003;**24**(9):699-706

[10] Palacios F, Campos M, Juarez JM, Cosgrove SE, Avdic E, Cánovas-Segura B, et al. A clinical decision support system for an antimicrobial stewardship program. In: HEALTHINF 2016-9th International Conference on Health Informatics, Proceedings. Rome: SciTePress; 2016. pp. 496-501

[11] Shortliffe EH. Computer-Based Medical Consultations: MYCIN. Elsevier; 1976

[12] Ma M, Shahar Y, Shortliffe EH. Clinical decision-support systems. Biomedical Informatics. 2006;**30**:698-736

[13] Kuperman GJ, Gardner RM, Pryor TA. HELP: A Dynamic Hospital Information System. Computers and Medicine. New York, NY: Springer; 1991

[14] Evans RS, Pestotnik SL, Classen DC, Clemmer TP, Weaver LK, Orme JF, et al. A computer-assisted management program for antibiotics and other antiinfective agents. New England Journal of Medicine. 1998;**338**(4):232-238

[15] Kahn MG, Sa S, Fraser VJ, Dunagan WC. An expert system for culture-based infection control surveillance. In: Proceedings of the Annual Symposium on Computer Applications in Medical Care. 1993. pp. 171-175

[16] Doherty J, Noirot LA, Mayfield J, Ramiah S, Huang C, Dunagan WC, et al. Implementing GermWatcher, an enterprise infection control application.

In: AMIA Annual Symposium Proceedings. 2006. pp. 209-213

[17] Lamma E, Mello P, Nanetti A, Riguzzi F, Storari S, Valastro G. Artificial intelligence techniques for monitoring dangerous infections. IEEE Transactions on Information Technology in Biomedicine. 2006;**10**(1):143-155

[18] Lo YS, Liu CT. Development of a hospital-acquired infection surveillance information system by using service-oriented architecture technology. In: 2010 3rd International Conference on Computer Science and Information Technology. vol. 4. IEEE. 2010. pp. 449-453

[19] Lovis C, Colaert D, Stroetmann VN. DebugIT for patient safety—Improving the treatment with antibiotics through multimedia data mining of heterogeneous clinical data. Studies in Health Technology and Informatics. 2008;**136**:641-646

[20] Schober D, Boeker M, Bullenkamp J, Huszka C, Depraetere K, Teodoro D, et al. The DebugIT core ontology: Semantic integration of antibiotics resistance patterns. Studies in Health Technology and Informatics. 2010;**160**:1060-1064

[21] Teodoro D, Pasche E, Gobeill J, Emonet S, Ruch P, Lovis C. Building a transnational biosurveillance network using semantic web technologies: Requirements, design, and preliminary evaluation. Journal of Medical Internet Research. 2012;**14**(3):e73

[22] Leibovici L, Paul M, Nielsen AD, Tacconelli E, Andreassen S. The TREAT project: Decision support and prediction using causal probabilistic networks. International Journal of Antimicrobial Agents. 2007;**30**:93-102

[23] Adlassnig KP, Blacky A, Koller W. Artificial-intelligence-based hospital-acquired infection control. Studies in Health Technology and Informatics. 2009;**149**:103-110

[24] Steurbaut K, Colpaert K, Gadeyne B, Depuydt P, Vosters P, Danneels C, et al. COSARA: Integrated service platform for infection surveillance and antibiotic management in the ICU. Journal of Medical Systems. 2012;**36**:3765-3775

[25] Beaudoin M, Kabanza F, Nault V, Valiquette L. An antimicrobial prescription surveillance system that learns from experience. AI Magazine. 2014;**35**(1):15-25

[26] Evans RS, Olson JA, Stenehjem E, Buckel WR, Thorell EA, Howe S, et al. Use of computer decision support in an antimicrobial stewardship program (ASP). Applied Clinical Informatics. 2015;**6**(1):120-135

[27] Simões AS, Maia MR, Gregório J, Couto I, Asfeldt AM, Simonsen GS, et al. Participatory implementation of an antibiotic stewardship programme supported by an innovative surveillance and clinical decision-support system. Journal of Hospital Infection. 2018; **100**(3):257-264

[28] Sackett DL. Evidence-based medicine. In: Encyclopedia of Biostatistics. Chichester, UK: John Wiley & Sons, Ltd; 2005

[29] WASPSS Project: Wise Antimicrobial Stewardship Support System. Available from: http://www.um.es/waspss/ [Accessed: 17 July 2019]

[30] Cánovas-Segura B, Campos M, Morales A, Juarez JM, Palacios F. Development of a clinical decision support system for antibiotic management in a hospital environment. Progress in Artificial Intelligence. 2016;**5**(3):181-197

[31] Cánovas-Segura B, Morales A, Juarez JM, Campos M, Palacios F. A lightweight acquisition of expert rules for interoperable clinical decision support systems. Knowledge-Based Systems. 2019;**167**:98-113

[32] Canovas-Segura B, Zerbato F, Oliboni B, Combi C, Campos M, Morales A, et al. A process-oriented approach for supporting clinical decisions for infection management. In: 2017 IEEE International Conference on Healthcare Informatics (ICHI); IEEE. 2017. pp. 91-100

[33] Morales A, Campos M, Juarez JM, Canovas-Segura B, Palacios F, Marin R. A decision support system for antibiotic prescription based on local cumulative antibiograms. Journal of Biomedical Informatics. 2018;**84**(July):114-122

[34] Garcia-caballero H, Campos M, Juarez JM, Palacios F. Visualization in clinical decision support system for antibiotic treatment. In: Actas de la XVI Conferencia de la Asociación Española para la Inteligencia Artificial, CAEPIA 2015, Albacete, Noviembre 9–12, 2015. 2015. pp. 71-80

[35] Sendelbach S, Funk M. Alarm fatigue: A patient safety concern. AACN Advanced Critical Care. 2013;**24**(4): 378-386

[36] Leclercq R, Cantón R, Brown DFJ, Giske CG, Heisig P, Macgowan AP, et al. EUCAST expert rules in antimicrobial susceptibility testing. Clinical Microbiology and Infection. 2013;**19**(2): 141-160

[37] EUCAST Expert Rules Version 3.1. The European Committee on Antimicrobial Susceptibility Testing; 2016. Available from: http://www.eucast.org/fileadmin/src/media/PDFs/EUCAST_files/Expert_Rules/Expert_rules_intrinsic_exceptional_V3.1.pdf [Accessed: 28 August 2018]

[38] Cánovas-Segura B, Campos M, Morales A, Juarez JM, Palacios F. Clinical decision support using antimicrobial susceptibility test results. In: Luaces O, Gámez JA, Barrenechea E, Troncoso A, Galar M, Quintián H, et al., editors. Advances in Artificial Intelligence: 17th Conference of the Spanish Association for Artificial Intelligence, CAEPIA 2016, Salamanca, Spain, September 14–16, 2016. Proceedings. 2016. pp. 251-260

[39] Cánovas-Segura B, Morales A, Juarez JM, Campos M, Palacios F. Impact of expert knowledge on the detection of patients at risk of antimicrobial therapy failure by clinical decision support systems. Journal of Biomedical Informatics. 2019;**94**:103200

[40] IOM (Institute of Medicine). Clinical Practice Guidelines We Can Trust. Washington, DC: The National Academies Press; 2011

[41] Kish MA. Guide to development of practice guidelines. Clinical Infectious Diseases. 2001;**32**(6):851-854

[42] Cabana MD, Rand CS, Powe NR, Wu AW, Wilson MH, Abboud PAC, et al. Why don't physicians follow clinical practice guidelines? JAMA. 1999; **282**(15):1458

[43] Cánovas-Segura B, Morales A, Lopez Martinez-Carrasco A, Campos M, Juarez JM, López Rodríguez L, et al. Improving interpretable prediction models for antimicrobial resistance. In: 2019 IEEE 32nd International Symposium on Computer-Based Medical Systems (CBMS). IEEE. 2019. pp. 543-546

[44] Morales A, Cánovas-Segura B, Campos M, Juarez JM, Palacios F. Proposal of a big data platform for intelligent antibiotic surveillance in a hospital. In: Luaces O, Gámez JA, Barrenechea E, Troncoso A, Galar M, Quintián H, et al., editors. Advances in Artificial Intelligence: 17th Conference of the Spanish Association for Artificial Intelligence, CAEPIA 2016, Salamanca, Spain, September 14–16, 2016. Proceedings. 2016. pp. 261-270